THE
H·I·G·H
BLOOD PRESSURE
RELIEF
DIET

Also by Dr. James Scala:
The Arthritis Relief Diet

THE
H·I·G·H
BLOOD PRESSURE
RELIEF
DIET

Dr. JAMES SCALA

NAL BOOKS

NEW AMERICAN LIBRARY

A DIVISION OF PENGUIN BOOKS USA INC., NEW YORK
PUBLISHED IN CANADA BY
PENGUIN BOOKS CANADA LIMITED, MARKHAM, ONTARIO

NOTE TO THE READER

The ideas, procedures, and suggestions contained in this book are not intended as a substitute for consulting with your physician. All matters regarding your health require medical supervision.

For information address New American Library

Published simultaneously in Canada by Penguin Books Canada Limited

 NAL TRADEMARK REG. U.S. PAT. OFF. AND FOREIGN COUNTRIES
REGISTERED TRADEMARK—MARCA REGISTRADA
HECHO EN CHICAGO, U.S.A.

SIGNET, SIGNET CLASSIC, MENTOR, ONYX, PLUME, MERIDIAN and NAL BOOKS are published *in the United States* by New American Library, a division of Penguin Books USA Inc., 1633 Broadway, New York, New York 10019, *in Canada* by Penguin Books Canada Limited, 2801 John Street, Markham, Ontario L3R 1B4.

Library of Congress Cataloging-in-Publication Data

Scala, James, 1934–
    The high blood pressure relief diet / by James Scala.
        p.   cm.
    Includes index.
    ISBN 0-453-00630-2
    1. Hypertension—Diet therapy.   2. High-potassium diet.
3. Salt-free diet.   4. Low-fat diet.   I. Title.
RC685.H8S26   1988
616.1′320654—dc19   88-21047
                                                                                CIP

Designed by Guy Ramsey

First Printing, January, 1989

              4   5   6   7   8   9

PRINTED IN THE UNITED STATES OF AMERICA

Dedication

To Nancy . . . it's been a great cruise.

In 1957, we signed on together as "mates" for our voyage through life. Our cruise has been rewarding—five great children, Jim, Scott, Greg, Nancy, and Kim; a new daughter, Joan, and a granddaughter, Julianna—all beautiful. We've navigated through smooth seas, rough seas, and a few storms; but we reefed the sails and kept going to sunny skies.

With this book we have a new star to steer by. We can discover warm seas, new anchorages, and unknown shores. We'll still be young with opportunities to help others, to be better ourselves, and to enjoy the sunshine.

Contents

FOREWORD

High blood pressure, or hypertension, is certainly one of the most common and important disorders seen by physicians, especially cardiologists. If left undiagnosed or untreated, it markedly increases the risk of stroke, heart attack, and kidney disease. As Dr. Scala clearly explains, 9 out of every 10 cases of high blood pressure are primary or "essential" hypertension. Once secondary hypertension is ruled out, primary hypertension is relatively easy to diagnose. It takes just a few minutes for a health professional or even the person himself to measure blood pressure. If high blood pressure is detected, the next decision is how it should be treated, either with or without drugs.

As a practicing cardiologist for over twenty years, I have seen the pendulum swing away from drug therapy to non-drug therapy. I have always believed in the medical philosophy "primum non nocere," meaning "first do no harm." The non-pharmacologic (non-drug) therapy for mild to moderate hypertension includes lowering salt intake, weight reduction, exercise, and stress management. If done carefully and with proper knowledge, there is little or no risk of any harm from this behavior modification. On the other hand, drug therapies with either diuretics, beta-blockers, or vasodilators have small but definite side effects or risks.

Dr. Scala has explained in easily understandable terms the physiologic or scientific mechanisms of hypertension. He has then proceeded to make the argument for non-drug therapy. Much of this book also outlines practical routines and regimens for low dietary salt intake and a favorable sodium–potassium balance. I agree with him that a low salt diet is the cornerstone of non-drug therapy. One of the major

ix

problems has been how to reduce salt intake to therapeutic levels and still maintain adequate nutrition, and more important, compliance. The old "rice diet" consisting almost entirely of plain rice for every meal effectively lowers blood pressure by its low salt content of around 200 milligrams per day. However, it was almost impossible to maintain this severe restriction for any period of time unless in a clinic or hospital setting. The "high blood pressure relief diet" is a safe, effective and more practical method. Dr. Scala carefully presents a practical regimen along with palatable recipes which can be followed throughout all phases of life, especially with increasing age when high blood pressure is more common.

In my medical practice, I have always believed that patients should take an active part in maintaining their health. This can be accomplished or at least aided in almost any illness. The treatment of high blood pressure along with avoidance of smoking and reducing high cholesterol and dietary fat are the major risk modifications to prevent heart attacks and coronary artery disease. In this book, *The High Blood Pressure Relief Diet*, Dr. Scala has presented in readable form both the theory and practice of blood pressure control. He has an excellent scientific background in nutrition dating back to his Ph.D. degree in Biochemistry from Cornell University. He has published numerous articles in scientific journals and has worked in nutrition research since obtaining his doctorate degree. He also practices what he preaches in maintaining a healthy lifestyle. His easily comprehended writing style along with many interesting caveats makes for informative and delightful reading. This is a superb book for the novice as well as those more knowledgeable about hypertension. I learned from it and thoroughly enjoyed it. It is an excellent book in the field of preventive medicine, which is the "best medicine."

John L. Penny, M.D.
Director, Cardiac Catheterization Laboratory
Director, Division of Cardiology
Valley Hospital, Ridgewood, New Jersey

ACKNOWLEDGMENTS

I could never have written this book without the help, support, and encouragement of some exceptional people. I owe them my sincere thanks and gratitude.

Al Zuckerman, my agent, stood behind me when the issue was in doubt. He is truly a man of integrity.

Alexia Dorszynski, like Al, believed in the concepts in the book. She was always there to help and answer questions. Her interest and guidance is the mark of an ideal editor. I will watch as her star continues to rise.

Katie Rosenthal has been the most pleasant, positive, supportive editor any author could ever hope to have. I hope I can do another book with Katie's guiding hand and spirit.

A special word of thanks to John Penny, M.D., an outstanding physician and a truly humane man, for reading the manuscript and then supporting it without reservation. I am grateful for his encouragement and kind words.

My daughter, Kim, was a real inspiration. Her bright, cheerful smile, willingness to help, and understanding during long hours will always be cherished and remembered.

Louise Morris, my sister, has always been supportive of my dream.

Finally, my partner and wife, Nancy. When we took our vows thirty-one years ago, it was for better or for worse, but I never told her it would also be "for lunch." My deepest love and thanks.

To all these people I extend my heartfelt thanks and sincere appreciation.

Section One

High Blood Pressure Basics and Origins

Prologue

Health Insurance vs. Sickness Insurance

Our medical system uses drug therapy as the first line of treatment. There are many reasons for this. After all, people have always sought simple, quick remedies for illness. And why not, who wants to be sick? What began with folk remedies progressed to the antibiotics of the 1940s, which rivaled the miracles described in the New Testament. But that was just the beginning. Pharmacology has since progressed to almost every type of illness and disease, bringing renewed health to millions of people.

As our medical and hospital costs have soared, health insurance has gained a necessary place. It usually pays for all medications and drugs. Indeed, "red tape" is cut quickly in the system if you have a well-defined illness and can take a drug for treatment. But "health insurance" has become a misnomer; it's really "sickness cost insurance" that permits people to use health professionals more effectively. It doesn't insure that you'll be healthy.

Insurance eliminates most of the financial burdens of illness, but it has created two other serious problems. If a dietary alternative exists, there seldom is an effective way within the system to compensate for regular individual or group counseling by an independent dietician or nutritionist. Perhaps one or even two visits would be partially paid for by the insurance, but the red tape for the patient and

3

the doctor would soon convince the doctor not to attempt diet therapy. Since the insurance won't pay, the uninformed can easily assume diet therapy is inferior or somehow not "legal." A passive patient doesn't participate in the restoration and maintenance of his own health; he leaves it in the hands of others.

Something has been sacrificed by this system. All drugs, no matter how mild, have side effects. Drugs for high blood pressure are no different. Possible side effects range from excessive excretion of potassium, to impotence, loss of sex drive, and many other complaints, including depression. If medication were the only way, the benefits would justify the costs in both money and side effects.

With high blood pressure, however, drug therapy is not the only way. In about 11% of all cases, high blood pressure is secondary to another illness and medical interventions or drug therapy is "the only way." Virtually 100% of the remaining 89% will not only benefit from a dietary and lifestyle approach, but 75% to 85% of them will never need to use drugs again if they continue to follow a prudent diet and lifestyle. Think on that for a moment . . . that figure translates to about 22 million of the over 35 million high blood pressure sufferers. These people can control, indeed eliminate completely, the symptoms of their illness and lead normal lives without drugs. And the remaining 13 million people can so effectively stabilize their illness that their need for drugs would be reduced to a minimum.

So you ask, if it's so easy, why don't we do it?

I like to think it's because people, including their physicians, simply don't know about the possibility, but I know it's more than that. People like to go to the doctor and get a problem "fixed" quickly and easily with a pill or an injection. Health insurance makes it easier if that's the outcome, because it usually accepts the cost of the prescription. And too often, the doctor doesn't present the alternative, if he knows one exists.

But I don't blame the doctor. I spoke in a symposium on

high blood pressure at a medical school. Of course, I advocated diet, and one of the debaters, a truly fine physician on the faculty, gave an argument that is tough for me to put down. It went like this:

"Dr. Scala, I applaud your efforts with diet, but I can't get my patients to take their medication more than 60% of the time. How well do you think they will comply with a diet program? I can't risk it." In that statement he said it all.

This book tells you about an obligation to yourself. You must actively participate in the restoration and maintenance of your own health. It's your body. The rewards are great—health without the need to take drugs. Our understanding of high blood pressure is so close to complete that changes in diet, lifestyle, and behavior can do it for most people. And that is what this book is all about. It simply tells you how.

Everyone now has a choice. The dietary and lifestyle programs in this book cannot cause harm and can only help. Enlist your doctor's support. He can tell you if you're making progress and suggest what form of exercise may be right for you. But most of all, his involvement and his recognition of the results will be like seeds sown in fertile soil, helping bring forth a return to basic concepts and an awareness that people can help themselves.

As success accumulates, another influence will be realized —a new "health insurance policy" for you. What we call "health insurance" is really insurance that compensates for the cost of sickness. True "health insurance" is the message of this book. It tells you how to really insure your health so you can live life to the fullest and take advantage of the bounty this beautiful world has to offer.

Chapter One

The Who, What, When of High Blood Pressure

Who

Over 20 percent of all adults in America over age 35 have high blood pressure (hypertension). That comes to more than 35 million people. It seems to affect men and women equally and is slightly more prevalent among the black population. So, if you've got high pressure, you're not alone.

What

Blood pressure is measured by wrapping a band, called a cuff, around your arm, pumping it up, and listening below the cuff for two sounds as the pressure in the cuff is released. The first sound is a thump, thump, thump of the heartbeat; that gives a high number, the systolic blood pressure. The second sound is a steady flow when the pressure in the cuff is low enough to let the blood flow smoothly; that is the diastolic pressure.

Blood pressure is expressed as a ratio of systolic over diastolic. For example, your systolic might be 140 and your diastolic 85. That's simply expressed by the physician as 140/85 and is accepted as borderline hypertension.

In subsequent chapters, we'll discuss blood pressure in

more detail. For now, if your blood pressure is regularly 140/85, you should take steps to get it down. You should strive to keep it below 130/80.

When

When your diastolic blood pressure is consistently over 90, you've got hypertension. In my opinion, you should follow the plan in this book when it's consistently over 80 and absolutely when it's over 85. You might get the idea from this that hypertension is not a clearly defined illness; you're correct. At a diastolic of 90, your doctor will say you've got it! But between 80 and 85, he might not even say "watch it," and from 85 to 89, he might say it's "high normal." I propose that anything over 80 should be treated seriously.

In subsequent chapters we'll discuss this in much more detail, but this helps to identify my concern.

Insidious Onset

People usually learn they have high blood pressure in one of two ways. It either seems to develop under the physician's watchful eye, or it's "there." Let me explain and you might see yourself in these situations.

In one case, you go in for a checkup and the doctor or nurse takes your blood pressure a few times, asks you if you've been tense lately, or under stress, and tells you to drop by in a week or so to have your blood pressure taken again. You're assured that it's nothing to worry about; they're just checking. The next time it's still elevated and you're asked if there's a history of high blood pressure in your family. It might even be suggested that you lose a few pounds, cut back on salt, and cut back on alcohol. It often continues this way for months, up to a year or two before it's decided that you've got high blood pressure.

In contrast, the doctor or nurse takes your blood pressure a couple of times and starts asking if high blood pressure runs in your family. You find out all at once that you've got high blood pressure. Indeed, it could be 140/93 or even higher, and there's no doubt in your doctor's mind.

In both extremes, you feel fine, not a sick day in your life. That's why we call high blood pressure the "silent killer." High blood pressure does have symptoms, as you'll learn in subsequent chapters, but they are so minor, so insidious, that they become "normal" to you and you never realize you are developing a serious disease.

You Can Do It

Blood pressure control without drugs is within your personal power. But you must make a personal commitment to yourself to gain complete control of your health. This book tells you how to regain control, restore your blood pressure to normal, and maintain a healthy life with increased longevity. If you follow the food plan and lifestyle programs in this book you will succeed. I promise!

Once you experience and measure the results of your commitment, you will ask yourself why you didn't start sooner. And what started as a diet program will become a welcome new way of life. You will be proud of yourself and set an example for others, especially the next generation.

"Let Food Be Thy Medicine"

Almost 2,500 years ago, Hippocrates, the Greek physician we call the father of modern medicine, made this profound statement. He was speaking of two possibilities. The first is preventive and the second is therapeutic. If Hippocrates could have the advantages of modern medical education, his words would be even more appropriate today than they were in 450 B.C. when he based them on his observation of typical illness of the time. His teaching has special meaning for sufferers of high blood pressure because food is most of what it's all about. Let a conversation I had tell it all.

Frank's Story

Frank is a very successful business man, age 51 at this writing, about 5'11" tall, and definitely overweight, at just over 200 pounds. But to his wife, friends, and family, he only needs to "lose a few pounds." Their attitude doesn't help. Frank has high blood pressure. He is now on medication that he must take daily—and he does about 60% of the time—for life. Our discussion went like this.

"When my doctor decided I had high blood pressure, he asked me what I wanted to do. Imagine that, *he asked me!*" Frank expected to be told, not asked.

I commented that his doctor sounded very much ahead of his time, because the control of high blood pressure is, in fact, the patient's decision.

Frank went on, "He gave me a diet that had me eliminate many of the foods I was eating. He said I'd have to lose 15 to 20 pounds." I asked about the diet.

"It wasn't hard to follow, because it simply cut out many processed foods and increased vegetables. And I had to stop salt, alcohol, use a food supplement, and start to exercise."

"Did it work?" I asked.

"Yes. On my next visit, one month later, the blood pressure was slightly high, the high end of normal," he said.

"Had you lost any weight?"

"Yes. I only lost about five pounds," he quickly added, "and I felt better."

For his exercise, he had purchased an exercise bicycle.

Obviously, Frank had achieved what his doctor had hoped for and what Hippocrates taught 2,500 years ago. So, what happened? Let Frank tell it.

"I didn't mind the diet for a while, but there are some foods I like to eat."

"Like what?" I questioned.

"Well, I go out to breakfast with friends and business associates. And I like linguista (a type of Portuguese sausage) with my order of eggs. I just started doing that again." He quickly added, "And I didn't have time to exercise because of the breakfast meetings."

"Was that all?" I was puzzled because I know there are ways to get around the linguista.

"Well, I started to have wine with lunch again, especially when I was with clients."

"And," I added, "the weight started coming back."

"Yes," he nodded and added, "it came back quickly and the blood pressure with it . . . I could tell."

I completed another confession for him. "I can't exercise in the evening myself. Could you do it?" He shook his head no. So he had stopped exercising altogether.

By the time Frank got to his four-month follow-up, his doctor observed that he was now back in the "high" range and would have to go on medication. But his doctor urged him to keep following the diet. Frank does make a half-hearted attempt regularly . . . sort of like the smoker who promises to quit between each cigarette and quits between each pack.

I urged Frank to follow the diet again and add an exercise program. He promptly followed what I do and purchased an exercise device that simulates cross-country skiing. He used it about ten times and now it sits, like new, in an extra bedroom. Whenever I ask Frank how his exercise plan is coming, the conversation goes like this:

"I get this low back pain."

I ask the obvious. "What did your doctor say about it?"

"It's not serious; mostly sore muscles from being out of shape."

Again, the obvious. "Why don't you start slow, try ten minutes a day for several weeks, and then work up?"

"I'm going to."

Silently, to myself, I add, "And the next time I see you, it will be exactly the same."

An Analysis of Frank

Frank is indeed one of the most fortunate men alive. He has a doctor who is a student of the teachings of Hippocrates, but with a modern medical education. He uses chronic medication as a last approach. But more important, he told his patient the truth: that it was up to him. Did Frank accept the responsibility? No!

In our conversations everything came out.

Proper diet is necessary; Frank has to learn to reduce his sodium intake and increase potassium, striving for the magic ratio of three times (or more) as much potassium as sodium. Indeed, he can eat linguista in moderation once in a while, as long as he compensates with other foods. The same with the wine—once in a while is okay.

Frank needs to lose weight. Over 200 pounds is too much for a sedentary 5'11" man. About 180 to 185 should be an upper limit, unless he hardens those soft muscles. He is one of those fortunate people who, if they lose just a little weight, about 5% of body weight, quickly reduce their blood pressure. So why not do it? Lack of motivation. In that, Frank is typical. I only hope the motivation isn't his first heart attack.

Exercise is essential. Frank is like many of us. He sees that I use an exercise device that simulates strenuous cross-country skiing and thinks if it keeps me in shape all he has to do is get one and follow suit. It's not that simple. I've maintained an exercise program for over twenty years and only recently bought this expensive device so I could get my exercise, watch the TV news, and escape jogging in the rain on narrow roads. There is no "ideal" exercise, but if it works for me, it's "ideal" for me. Frank should have started a walking program. Or, if he likes cross-country skiing, he should have started slowly; say ten minutes at an easy pace for a month and work his way up. But no, he wanted unrealistic, quick results. Life is simply not that way.

Frank's doctor, while certainly on the right track, didn't go far enough. He should have made Frank purchase this book if it had existed and have him send in the weekly results of his weight and blood pressure measurements.

What This Book Will Do For You

You can gain a new lease on life if you give yourself a chance. This book will tell you how. High blood pressure is your body's way of saying you're doing something wrong and it's not just one thing. It's a combination of diet, lifestyle, and, to some extent, heredity. That's right. Who you chose for parents and maybe even more important, grandparents, affects your health. But that's not an excuse, because with blood pressure, heredity can be overcome!

Since no one can do anything about choice of parents, we'll simply overcome those effects by diet and lifestyle. In these pages a plan will unfold. This plan helps you to regain control of your diet, develop some new aspects of lifestyle, and even use some relaxation techniques. All I ask is that you do it one day at a time, working toward realistic goals.

Someday, not that far off, if you reflect back, you'll realize that you have exchanged new habits for old. You'll realize that your life is full, you can smell the roses a little better, taste an apple more keenly, sleep more soundly, wake up with greater bounce, work or play longer hours, and provide an example to your friends, loved ones, and the next generation so they can avoid high blood pressure altogether.

Will It Work For Everyone?

Yes! To some extent.

You may think the "to some extent" sounds like the proverbial TV ad with its safe caveat, or the fine print in a contract. I'll explain what I mean.

Some people with high blood pressure, less than 15%, always require some medication. It's called pharmacologic therapy. But diet even helps *them* dramatically! It reduces the amount of drugs these people require and stabilizes their illness. Diet and lifestyle can become the major factor in their defense.

High blood pressure, the silent killer, is such a serious problem that the government, through the National Institutes of Health, has a committee to deal with the issue. This joint national committee of health professionals presented its first report in 1984. In the words of the joint national committee, "These [diet] approaches have particular relevance for patients with mild hypertension [high blood pressure], but have been shown to be of value in patients with more severe hypertension receiving pharmacologic therapy." Indeed, what the government is saying is that you will benefit, even if you are among the 15% who cannot get off medication.

Is It Easy?

I think it is! All but one step . . . the first one.

There is one part of any journey that is never easy— overcoming procrastination. Procrastination is simply mental inertia, similar to the physical inertia described by Isaac Newton. An object at rest tends to stay at rest! Don't do what Frank did . . . put off until tomorrow . . . or until his backache is gone . . . start now! Take a long walk, look at some flowers, some children, some birds singing; just don't stop for an ice cream or a drink. You can stop for an apple, though.

If you will give yourself a chance, someday soon you'll look back and wonder, "Why didn't I do it sooner?" And you'll want to know why more people don't do it.

Believe me, it is easy. I've seen too many people succeed.

Am I Too Old?

You're never too old! Read about Claire.

Claire came to me after a lecture I gave. She is a beautiful woman over 70 years old. My lecture that evening was on human longevity. The message was that with a little effort we can extend life expectancy 30% simply by applying the knowledge we already have. My message touched her.

She wanted to know if she could reduce her blood pressure by diet, and get off the medication she was taking. I gave her an emphatic yes! I added that it would require hard but pleasant work on her part. Her first task was to start to lose about 30 pounds and get on the program in this book. I received the following letter about six months later.

Dear Dr. Scala:

I've done it! My doctor says I don't need the medication anymore. My blood pressure is a slightly high normal. He wants me to have it checked regularly, but unless I backslide, I won't need medication ever again.

Claire goes on in her letter giving me all the credit. I don't deserve it. She did it by herself. All I did was set some short-term goals for her and tell her how to select her food and what to cut out. She did the rest. She proved for all of us that chronological age has nothing to do with the body's ability to improve. And by the way, her life expectancy has increased because of what she accomplished.

Are You Alone?

I have the privilege of speaking to folks all over the world. I like to speak to them about improving the quality and quantity of their lives. After all, everyone wants to live longer and live better. In the context of longevity, high blood pressure demands serious attention for two reasons. First, it is a major epidemic in every affluent country, affects over 35 million people in the U.S., and costs over $19 billion annually for medication alone. Second, blood pressure is unique because 89% can be controlled by diet and lifestyle. The remaining 11% that can't be completely controlled by diet and lifestyle can be significantly reduced.

The Silent Epidemic

Using the criteria established by the joint committee on detection and treatment of high blood pressure, about 20% of Americans over the age of 35 have high blood pressure. Here's another way to visualize that statistic.

About 50% of our population is over age 35; that's about 120 million people. Since 20% have high blood pressure, and about another 10% have it but have not been diagnosed, about one out of every four adults over 35 has high blood pressure.

About 35 million people have been diagnosed with high blood pressure. Most estimates state that over 25 million more people have high blood pressure but have not been diagnosed because it is largely without symptoms. But worse, a survey of people 65 and older shows that about 75% of them have high blood pressure. Since about 11% of the population is over 65, that means about 20 million folks who should be enjoying the golden years they've worked for are dealing with an illness that can be prevented and controlled by diet and lifestyle.

Look at it another way. Suppose you're sitting in a theater, a church, or in some other crowd. Count off about ten adults you estimate to be 35 or older. Of the ten you count, two will almost certainly have high blood pressure and a third will be so close that 50% of doctors would say he has the disease. If the group is skewed higher in age, the number with high blood pressure will be even greater.

You might ask, "If high blood pressure is so bad and so many people have it, why don't we have campaigns to stamp it out?"

We do! The problem is that no one dies of high blood pressure because it forms the foundation for many other illnesses that are fatal. In fact, many people don't even know they have it. It's called the "silent killer" because it often goes undetected. So, National High Blood Pressure Month, May, comes and goes every year and only people like me take notice. We notice it because we know what it does to people and families. And we know that it doesn't need to exist in any but a very few.

The Silent Killer

People who have high blood pressure die younger, but high blood pressure doesn't kill directly. It does contribute directly to the development of other diseases that are very deadly indeed. And if those diseases don't kill, the victim often leads an impaired life, sometimes seeing death as a welcome relief.

High blood pressure reduces life expectancy. This relationship is so clearly established that I can say with certainty that someone with a diastolic blood pressure of 80 has a death rate slightly above normal and people with a diastolic of 100 (not an uncommon level) have twice the normal death rate. The probability of an early death goes up dramatically from there.

But people with high blood pressure usually die from a list of other disastrous illnesses. These deadly illnesses include stroke, heart attack, and kidney failure. High blood pressure also reduces the quality of life because, among other things, it can cause the loss of eyesight. Drugs that are used to control high blood pressure often cause depression, loss of sexual capacity, and other debilitating side effects.

People with high blood pressure pay more for life insurance—if they can get it. Heart failure, the loss of the heart's ability to pump sufficient blood, develops in 75% of people with high blood pressure. And what's worse is that once heart failure is detected, only 50% of the victims survive five years.

But there's more to the blood pressure–health relationship. The factors that cause high blood pressure, including overweight, high-salt diet, and excess fat of the wrong kinds, contribute to other problems, including heart disease, cancer, osteoporosis, and others.

To You I Throw the Torch

So you can see why I urge people to take control of their lives. Reduce blood pressure through diet. The benefits will not only eliminate an insidious illness, but the new habits you develop will reduce your risk of heart disease, stroke, cancer, kidney disease, and even osteoporosis. In fact, the new habits can increase your life expectancy up to 30%. An increase of 30% might seem remote at this time, but it will have infinitely more meaning as you get older. Also, think of the anguish and hardship your premature death can bring to those you love.

Start now. This is a good time to resolve that you will take a nice walk every day. It doesn't have to be a jog, but I hope someday it will be. Just make the walk brisk and don't stop for about thirty minutes. Do it every day. As the pages of this book unfold, you'll learn just how easy it is to gain a new lease on a longer life without medication.

Chapter Two

High Blood Pressure Basics

Our Marvelous Vascular System

Our body is a marvelous system that is at once complex and wonderfully simple. It consists of about 50 trillion (50 followed by 12 zeros) individual cells divided into many tissues and organs that are divided further into systems. Each cell and each organ has a very definite purpose. The organs that concern us here include the skin, heart, lungs, kidneys, and some glands. The systems involved are the cardiovascular and excretory systems. Most tissues, especially muscle tissue and vascular tissue, are involved in high blood pressure. It would, however, require an anatomy text to identify all the organs, tissues, and systems that make the human body work.

Each individual cell requires many nutrients, some of which we don't fully understand. Oxygen is the most important nutrient. As nutrients are metabolized, waste products, the most abundant of which is carbon dioxide, must be removed. The cardiovascular system, a specialized complex organ system, is responsible for the distribution of nutrients to each cell and removal of wastes from each cell. It consists of a central pumping station (the heart, with the arterial system) to carry the nutrient-laden blood, including oxygen, from the heart to every tissue and cell. Its second part is the venous system, to carry blood laden with wastes, including carbon dioxide, back to be recycled after cleansing by the lungs and kidneys. The lungs remove the carbon dioxide and the kidneys remove the other wastes.

By comparing the heart to a pumping station, it is easy to understand why pressure enters the discussion. Like any other fluid pump, the heart pushes the blood around with a force we call blood pressure. Because the heart pushes the blood into the arterial system on a single stroke, two pressures are important. The higher, systolic pressure, is the force generated when the blood is pushed into the arteries, and the lower, the diastolic, is the pressure that remains when the pumping chamber of the heart, the left ventricle, relaxes to fill with another volume of blood in preparation for the next push.

Bright red oxygen-laden blood is pumped by the heart into the largest artery, the aorta. The aorta then branches into smaller and smaller arteries. Think of the system as a tree: the trunk, which branches into twigs on a tree, which get smaller and go to each leaf. Similarly the arteries go into very small arterioles and to microscopic capillaries that infiltrate every tissue carrying oxygen and nutrients so they can enter each cell. Waste products then diffuse into other capillaries that form up in larger and larger branches, the way small streams form a river, to return the waste-laden venous blood, dark with carbon dioxide, to be cleansed and returned to the heart to be pumped out for another voyage through the system.

The arterioles and veins that bring blood to and from the muscles and skin constitute what we call the peripheral circulatory system. In addition to bringing oxygen and nutrients to the cells and removing carbon dioxide and waste materials, this system helps regulate body temperature. Peripheral blood flow helps regulate temperature by either increasing blood flow to the surface so heat is radiated into the environment, or restricting blood flow so heat is conserved. During exercise, for example, blood flow is increased not only to meet nutrient demands but also to radiate away heat. Conversely, in a cold environment, blood flow to the surface is reduced to maintain body temperature.

Normal Blood Pressure

Normal adult blood pressure, on average, is 120 systolic and 80 or less diastolic, simply expressed as 120 over 80. Individually, the numbers are actually expressed as millimeters of mercury; when expressed as a fraction such as 120/80, they have no dimensions because they are simply relative. Blood pressure is no longer always measured as millimeters of mercury. However, a column of mercury is actually used to precisely calibrate the instruments, making the unit meaningful, and physicians still often use devices that have columns of mercury.

"Normal" actually relates to the blood pressure of the average, healthy individual of the age category in question. It can vary rather widely; for example, my blood pressure is usually 110 over 70 or less, and sometimes it is as low as 100/60. On occasion, when I'm very nervous or active, it soars to 130/90. A rule of thumb teaches that systolic should be 100 plus your age, up to age 20, and diastolic should be 40 less than systolic. So, for our purposes, normal is 120/80. But recognize that a little higher or lower is still within the bounds of normal.

How Is Blood Pressure Determined?

Blood pressure is the combined product of the amount of blood that is actually pumped, the rate of the pumping, and the total resistance that it must overcome. In medical terminology, we say that blood pressure is the product of cardiac output and total peripheral resistance. It follows that there are two major determinants of blood pressure: the heart output and the factors that restrict blood flow. Let's take it a step at a time.

Heart (Cardiac) Output

Cardiac output is the result of stroke volume, or the amount of blood expelled by each contraction of the pumping chamber, multiplied by the actual number of beats per minute. Neither the arterial system nor the venous system is meant to be a rigid conduit. On the contrary, each should be flexible and capable of distending and contracting. By distending or contracting, the venous system becomes a dynamic reservoir that can determine how much blood from each stroke is returned to the heart. If the venous system is rigid and constricted, the return volume will be large. Consequently, each stroke must expel a large volume. It follows that this can elevate blood pressure simply because the heart has a greater volume to expel. Put another way, it's got a larger task to perform.

Total Peripheral Resistance

You can figure this factor out quite easily, but let me walk you through it so we'll be on common ground. Once blood is pumped from the heart, the resistance to flow is determined by three factors: the flowability or viscosity of the blood, the elasticity or flexibility of the arteries, and the number and diameter of the arterioles.

Viscosity is a way of expressing the resistance of liquid to flow. For example, on a cold day in January, molasses, honey, or motor oil is thick and "viscous"; it doesn't flow easily. In contrast, in July, it runs like water; it has a low viscosity. So blood viscosity describes blood's ability to flow. Blood with low viscosity flows more easily than that with high viscosity.

"Elasticity of the arterial walls" is an expression that describes their ability to stretch. They can be like a set of rigid pipes or flexible and stretchable like a rubber hose that handles surges in water pressure by giving and relaxing. The less rigid the arteries, the lower the blood pressure will be.

Diameter and abundance of the arterioles is the third and usually most dominant factor that determines blood pressure. Back to the analogy of the tree and its twigs: The larger the twigs, the more easily sap can flow to the leaves. The same with the arterioles. The arterioles that bring blood to the muscles and skin make up the peripheral blood flow. In technical terms, the more dilated the arterioles, and the more flexible the venous system, the lower the blood pressure will be.

In conclusion, total peripheral resistance consists of the "viscosity" of the blood, the "elasticity" of the arteries, and the number, size, and state of the arterioles. All three factors contribute to high blood pressure. It follows that by reducing blood viscosity and causing the arterioles and arteries to relax, blood pressure can be reduced. It will be reduced because total peripheral resistance will be less. Therefore, the same functions that cause the problem can be used to eliminate the problem.

How High Is "Too High"?

A father-and-son team of physicians, the Janeways, reported in 1913 that about 11% of their patients had systolic blood pressure over 165 millimeters of mercury. Significantly, they also noted that these patients didn't live as long as those whose systolic pressure was not so high. It is now accepted by all health agencies worldwide that the more elevated the blood pressure, the greater the risk of an early death from a number of illnesses, ranging from stroke to kidney failure, so it's important to diagnose the presence of high blood pressure and to deal with it effectively.

In 1984, the National Committee on High Blood Pressure published its conclusions in the *Archives of Internal Medicine*. Since diastolic blood pressure is considered the most critical, they emphasized it in their report. But they were also very specific about systolic blood pressure. They classified blood pressure as follows:

Classification of Blood Pressure

Range in Millimeters of Mercury Diastolic BP	*Category of Hypertension*
Less than 85	Normal Blood Pressure
85 to 89	High Normal
90 to 104	Mild Hypertension
105 to 114	Moderate Hypertension
115 or higher	Severe Hypertension

Systolic BP Diastolic BP Less Than 90	
Less than 140	Normal
140 to 159	Borderline Isolated Systolic Hypertension
160 or more	Isolated Systolic Hypertension

Ranges of blood pressure and severity of hypertension bring two things to mind. Blood pressure doesn't go from normal to severe hypertension overnight. Indeed, it creeps up slowly. Diastolic pressure between 80 and 84 millimeters of mercury should be considered the "warning" zone where diet should change. The clue to this zone's seriousness is that insurance companies take it into account when selling a life insurance policy.

Two Types of High Blood Pressure

About 10% of cases of high blood pressure are the result of a specific problem, such as kidney disease, an adrenal tumor, or constriction of the major artery (the aorta), to name a few. When such a cause is identified, the hypertension is called "secondary," because it is the by-product of another illness and when that illness is corrected, the hypertension usually disappears.

The other type of hypertension, known as "essential hypertension," affects about 90% of people with high blood pressure. It's what we call common high blood pressure. The specific cause is actually unknown. It is usually the result of many factors, such as heredity, overweight, poor diet, and lack of fitness, to name a few. Essential hypertension is what we will deal with in this book.

Symptoms

High blood pressure is called the silent killer because it usually goes undiagnosed. People with the problem may never know they have it. One day you have a physical, perhaps for insurance, or visit the doctor for some other reason; he takes your blood pressure and it's there. Indeed, if your diastolic blood pressure went from 70 one day to 105 the next, you'd know it. You would get the symptoms all at once. But it doesn't happen like that. It creeps up, often over many years, and your body adjusts to the change; you feel "normal" all the time until that day your doctor or the nurse says, "Your blood pressure's too high!" and gently starts talking of losing weight, cutting salt, and trying some medication. But some symptoms do appear that can be warning signs in the early stages. If you look back, you will probably remember some of them.

Headaches, especially in the morning
Ringing in the ears

Unexplained dizziness
Spontaneous nosebleeds
Depression without apparent cause
Blurred vision
Tension when there is no cause
Flushing of the face; redness
Fainting spells

An Inherited Tendency

Just about every aspect of our health has a heredity component. The influence of heredity ranges from personality and behavior to the probability of getting cancer. So what about high blood pressure? Until the recent decade, we had thought that high blood pressure was largely an inherited trait. And it wasn't surprising to identify families in which there were people with high blood pressure in each generation. In addition, Lewis Dahl, a scientist I had the pleasure of knowing, bred a strain of laboratory animals with hereditary high blood pressure. But today we know more.

Not a Certainty

Many populations simply don't seem to get high blood pressure. In those populations, about 1% or 2% usually get it, but in those cases, it's usually due to an identifiable illness and in our terminology is secondary hypertension. (If the illness is cleared up, the blood pressure returns to normal.)

Since these people in their native environment don't get primary or essential hypertension, we could erroneously assume they are resistant to high blood pressure. But, if we follow people from these populations into our society and keep track of their health, we observe that about one third of them will develop high blood pressure, the kind we call essential or primary hypertension. Therefore, we conclude that there's an inherited tendency triggered by something in the environment. Alcoholism is like that; the tendency is there in some people, just waiting for the right circumstances and booze to get it going.

With blood pressure, the environmental factor is food. After all, the environment inside our body is controlled by us with food and drink. In the case of essential hypertension we become what we eat. The difference between our food and the food of the native populations I spoke of is natural versus man-made. As a result of processing, the American diet has changed; let me give you some examples that I have summarized from USDA data.

In 1900, when our diet was largely unprocessed, we consumed 50 grams of sugar daily; that's a little under 2 ounces. And we added 35 grams ourselves. For example, on cereal (porridge in those days) and in coffee, etc., only 15 grams, or 25%, was hidden in the food. Nowadays we consume about 120 to 130 grams daily, say 125 grams or 4½ ounces. Take a 6-ounce juice glass and fill it to about an inch from the top and that's how much sugar we consume daily per capita. But that's not all: about 75%, or 94 grams, is hidden in the food we eat. We only add 32 grams ourselves.

In 1900, we consumed about 25% of our calories as fat. From a man burning 2,500 calories daily, that was 70 grams daily, or about 2½ ounces; in practical terms, 2½ half pats of butter daily. Today we consume 42% of our calories as fat, or 116 grams for the same man. That's over 4 pats of butter. Think of all that fat clogging your arteries; worse yet, as a nice roll around your waist, because we don't get as much exercise as people did in 1900.

But the real villain for our purposes is salt. In 1900, the diet contained about 4½ grams of salt, and over 75% was added directly. Now we consume over 8 grams, and 75% is hidden; only 25% is added directly.

Another way to describe our present diet is that we live in a sea of sugar with islands made of fat, topped with trees of salt. Our diet has gotten out of control! Many people seem to do all right on this diet when they have youth on their side. But 75% of people over 65 have high blood pressure. And one out of five deaths over 65 are from a heart attack, stroke or related incident.

The natural diet is the diet that man evolved in and that shaped his metabolism. We are not equipped with the metabolic machinery to consume a diet with all that sugar, fat, and salt. And when we do consume it, problems develop.

Potassium–Sodium Balance

From Dahl's pioneering research, we know that sodium, and specifically salt, is a prime culprit in high blood pressure. Physicians speak of "salt-sensitive hypertensives." These are people who develop high blood pressure from too much salt. If they simply reduce their salt intake so the sodium content of their diet is less than about 800 milligrams, the high blood pressure usually disappears. But, a diet that reduces salt intake will be naturally higher in potassium, and now we know the dietary problem is more complex than just too much salt. Salt is still a major factor with many people, but for a majority, it's the balance between sodium and potassium that is crucial.

The K Factor

This balance between potassium and sodium and its impact on high blood pressure was the subject of a recent book by Dr. Richard D. Moore and Dr. George D. Webb entitled *The K Factor*. The K Factor is a way of describing a food, a meal, or an entire eating habit. A good K Factor would be 3 or greater. The figure is a ratio easily obtained by simply dividing the amount of potassium in a food by the amount of sodium in it. Let's look at a few typical foods:

Food	Sodium	Potassium	K-Factor
Apple	1	159	159.00
Avocado	21	1,097	52.00
Hot dog	461	71	0.15
Cornflakes	351	26	0.07
Roast beef (slice)	46	547	12.00
Corn	4	226	56.00
Apple pie (frozen)	298	73	0.24
Frozen meat loaf (5 ounces)	951	196	0.20

From the above table, it's easy to see that some foods, especially the natural ones, are high in potassium and low in sodium. Other foods, usually man-made, are high in sodium and low in potassium. Put another way, the K Factor of natural foods tends to be high, and in some man-made foods, it is very low.

About one third of the human population can't tolerate a diet that contains less than about two times as much potassium as sodium or a K Factor of two. Most of these same people apparently cannot tolerate the large amounts of sodium in our diet even if the K Factor remained above two.

Another group of high blood pressure sufferers is emerging. The high-renin hypertensives. The kidneys of these people produce excess amounts of an enzyme called renin that indirectly causes the arterioles to constrict and the kidneys to retain salt. Both effects will elevate the blood pressure. The renin can be blocked and then these people can handle the salt.

Other Factors

Once doctors and nutrition researchers understood that about one third of the population can't handle a dietary K

Factor of less than 3, we looked for other factors contributing to hypertension. Overweight turned out to be another major factor. Many people who are seriously overweight tend to develop high blood pressure. It's easy to see that The extra force necessary to get the blood through all that flab simply requires more pressure. This interpretation is overly simplistic, however, because another hormone, insulin, is involved. We'll explore it in detail in a later chapter, so for now, let the idea of extreme force stand. It follows that overweight people with high blood pressure only need return to normal weight and the blood pressure returns to normal. That's just about what we observe! In fact, the blood pressure usually drops more quickly than the weight. In one study at the Scripps Clinic, blood pressure dropped by about 12% when weight had dropped less than 5%. So, if the interpretation is oversimplistic, the results are fantastic!

There are also some people whose behavior maintains them in a type of "stress" that keeps them tense and causes blood pressure to elevate. We think of these people as Type A personalities. We'll discuss them later.

Is Heredity Final?

Absolutely not! Unequivocally, heredity is not even an excuse any longer. In high blood pressure, the hereditary tendency is not a firm trait like your eye color. Indeed, an inherited tendency simply is a warning flag that says "take care of your body and everything will be just fine." I like to put it in a more positive way. If you've inherited the tendency, you're lucky because you know the boundary lines within which you've got to live. No need for you to experiment and search; you're in control of your health!

Gene's Story

One morning after giving a speech on longevity in which blood pressure was a main point, I saw a member of the audience sitting alone for breakfast, so I asked to join them. He looked pensive, so I asked what thoughts were troubling him. I got Gene's story.

Everyone in his family has high blood pressure. He was on a medication—one I am very familiar with—that reduces sexual activity in men to zip!

I asked him what he was going to do about it. His reply made me seethe.

"Well, Doc, it's in my genes; there's nothing I can do." He looked sad. I asked if the drug was effective.

"Yes, it keeps the blood pressure right in line and I feel good."

"Are there any side effects?" I played dumb.

"Well, it cuts out my sex life." That was my cue. I asked him how a man his age (my age) could pass up the most pleasurable and intimate human experience without a fight. He gave the old "it's in my genes" story.

I told him that if he'd lose weight (about twenty-five pounds), follow the diet plan in this book, and start an exercise program, he could get off drugs and gain a new lease on life. Somehow I motivated him, because he started this program. And although he's no ball of fire, he is making progress. His weight is coming down, he doesn't require as much of a new, less potent medication, and there's more sparkle in his eye. I think some of his sexual capacity is restored. It makes me feel good.

So, if you have primary hypertension, common high blood pressure, and you think it's heredity, you're mistaken. If your doctor told you so, he's using obsolete information. All heredity means with high blood pressure is that you've got to work a little harder. Take your life a little more seriously until you develop the habits that will restore your health.

Type A Behavior

Some people seem to have personalities that predispose them toward high blood pressure and heart disease. They have particularly aggressive personalities and seem driven. We call these Type A personalities, and I will discuss them in detail later.

Bill's Story

Bill has a typical Type A personality and has high blood pressure, but for now, I want you to see his symptoms.

Bill is a typical type A executive. Already, at age 43, he is the president of a Fortune 500 company, and his star is still rising.

One day I went into his office and there was blood all over his shirt. Sue, his secretary, told me he had a nosebleed. Her eyes were wide with concern. I spoke to her and asked around, and determined that Bill has had nosebleeds quite often. Then a fortuitous event occurred. He was testing a blood pressure measuring device his company was thinking of selling and he called me one evening at home.

"Jim, I can't get this thing to work properly; could it be the batteries?"

I asked the obvious. "What reading does it give?"

"It keeps giving 140 over 89, and that's not right."

I told him that it looks to me that the instrument is correct; his blood pressure is high.

"It can't be; I don't have high blood pressure." And that was the end of our discussion.

Since our conversation, Bill's doctor has convinced him he's got hypertension. His father does also.

To make a long story short, Bill is now on an exercise program (he doesn't follow it), a low-salt diet (he tries to follow it), and medication (he takes it only 60% of the time).

I know and Bill knows that he didn't just start getting nosebleeds at age 43. When he admitted his problem to me one day, he confessed that he had been having nosebleeds off and on for years. Occasionally, people would comment that he looked flushed, or he'd get a dizzy spell. And, no matter what the occasion, Bill was tense. If Bill had started a diet and lifestyle program when his blood pressure was 125/85, he wouldn't be in the dilemma he is in today. But it is not too late; at age 43, his life expectancy is about 33 years. With that much productive life ahead of him, he should make them the healthiest of his life.

In this brief review you have become more aware of your cardiovascular system. This marvelous system usually functions so well that most of the time we don't even know of its existence, but when abused by diet and lifestyle, it often develops high blood pressure. These abuses include excess weight, dietary sodium, and a poor dietary K Factor; you control all of them. As you read this book, you will realize that by taking control of these factors, blood pressure will return to normal. More important, if your blood pressure is normal now, follow these concepts and it will never get high.

Chapter Three
Knowledge Can Set You Free

Know Yourself

Understand the origins of your own high blood pressure and you will be free. You will know that you can choose to control it by diet as much as possible, or, conversely, that you can choose to be passive and give your doctor total control with drugs. I believe that people armed with knowledge usually make the best choices. Knowledge seems to have its own benefit.

A Weight-Loss Study

I first noticed the benefit of having people learn about their health from a weight-loss study conducted at a leading medical school, where I lectured. Rather than put overweight people on a "diet," participants were given talks on food and nutrition, with emphasis on the causes of overweight, and were taught how to figure out the caloric content of food. During the study they were asked to keep a food diary and critique their food intake daily. A food diary is like any other daily record; however, it focuses on food. Researchers asked the participants to write a paragraph or two at the end of the day describing the quality of their food for the day.

Every person in the group lost weight. And they kept it off. I think the people in this study proved two points very clearly. Once they understood the basis of overweight, they shifted their eating habits toward reducing caloric intake. They selected foods that increased bulk and reduced fat and simple sugar. Those who had personal problems started to deal with them. More important, they never consciously went on a "diet" to lose weight. By understanding their eating habits, they were able, as motivated and informed adults, to take control and accomplish an objective that had eluded them for years.

Salt-Reduction Study

During one session at the same medical school the need for salt reduction in high blood pressure was emphasized. We know today that salt reduction is only part of the story. At various times during the program the participants would taste a low-salt soup for us and then add salt to taste. They didn't know that the amount of salt they used was accurately measured.

As the semester progressed, all the participants started to use significantly less salt. In fact, as the study ended, many were not adding any salt at all and were rating the soup quite highly. This was not an isolated incident; their food diaries indicated that the low-salt habit had pervaded all their eating.

From these studies and my work with people who have arthritis, asthma, and other chronic problems, I am sold on understanding. Understand how your body got to be the way it is and you've taken a giant step toward getting it back to normal. In the following pages you'll learn that there are many things you can do to return your blood pressure to normal. Some of these changes are easy, some not so easy, but simply knowing why you should be making them is a giant step.

Speak to Your Doctor First

If you purchased or were given this book, you either
have high blood pressure or have been told your blood
pressure is close to being high. I hope your doctor has
recommended that you work with diet, exercise, and lifestyle to avoid drugs. That's what this book is for. But you
need to get some things very clear from the doctor.

Is It Primary or Secondary?

Is your elevated blood pressure secondary? Secondary
high blood pressure means that you've got an illness and
the high blood pressure will probably clear when the illness
is cured. But the causative illness must be treated. This diet
will not hurt the illness and will help reduce the blood
pressure, but it should be followed under a doctor's guidance.

Is your elevated blood pressure primary, or essential,
hypertension? If it is, you've come to the right place. Now
tell your doctor that you want to work with diet. Ask him
to what extent your blood pressure is elevated; for example, is it at "high normal" or is it "seriously high"? In
either case, dietary work is fine, but at the serious end, you
may need medication while working with your diet and
lifestyle.

Are there any contraindications for you to eat a balanced
diet low in sodium and rich in potassium?

Are you diabetic? If so, can you reduce fat intake to less
than 35% of calories? Some diabetic specialists recognize a
small subgroup of patients they keep on a high-fat diet. Be
sure you're not one before you start.

Are there reasons why you should not lose weight (if
you're overweight) and enter a modest exercise program?

Ask for your doctor's or nurse's help in learning to take
your blood pressure and pulse.

How often does your doctor want to see you? For example, if you're on medication, as this dietary and lifestyle

program begins to work for you, the doctor is absolutely essential in setting the level of and reducing your medication. I hope you will be able to eliminate it and your doctor will be pulling for you.

Start a Food Diary

I'm always asked, "Should everyone use a food diary?" Yes! And for many good reasons.

Just as I want you to measure your pulse and blood pressure regularly, I want you to get in touch with the total you. And food is the major factor in returning your blood pressure to normal. We'll get into other factors, but none will be as effective as the food you eat.

So, what's a food diary? It's just about whatever you want to make it, but I'll explain what it should cover.

- *What* you ate and information about the serving size.
- *How much* salt and other condiments you used, including ketchup, pepper, salad dressing, meat sauces, etc.
- *All* snacks should be included, including mints, etc.
- *All* food supplements.
- *When* you ate it.
- *Why* you ate what you did. This can vary from hunger (e.g., breakfast) to being sociable (everyone else was drinking).
- *Critique* at the end of the day, in 25 words or less, how well you did. Give your opinion of the food you ate, the type of food, the amount, the reasons for eating it, and even the people you ate with. In short, evaluate your food day.

What to Look For

Your food diary will slowly become a part of your routine. It can tell you a great deal about yourself. For example, do you like natural foods? What processed foods do you use, and why? When do you eat, and most important, what? Are your snacks consistent with your meal patterns? For example, if you eat natural foods at meal time, are your snacks natural? How often do you use condiments such as salt, pepper, ketchup, sauce, and butter?

Get to know your eating habits and more important, how you can change them if necessary.

My Food Diary

There are no rules for a food diary, but over the years I've seen many that work and many that don't. I'll share what I think is the most practical type and explain why I think it works so well.

- Purchase a convenient, narrow-lined spiral notebook. I prefer the standard 8½ × 11, but I know people who use the next smaller size, 8 × 5. It's your choice.
- Rule off the pages into sections as follows: From the margin, mark columns at 1 inch, 3 inches, and 4 inches from the margin.
- Start each day with a new page. Learn to take each food day one at a time; put the date at the top of the page.
- The first column (at 1 inch) is marked "Time"; your first entry for example, might be 0700.
- The second column is marked "Food"; for example, oatmeal with milk.
- The third column is marked "Serving Size"; for example, ⅓ cup dry oatmeal, ½ cup milk.
- The fourth column is marked "Why Selected"; for example, "breakfast."

Let's see how this would look for a day's entry.

November 17, 1987

Time	Food	Serving Size	Why Selected
0700	Oatmeal with raisins & milk	⅓ cup ½ cup milk	Breakfast and I like it
0700	¼ cantaloupe		Tastes good and I like it
0700	2 cups tea	2 cups	Habit and lift
0700	1 Vita-Lea 1 B-complex 1 Vitamin C 500	N/A	Supplements are necessary in my opinion
1030	Cup of tea	1 cup	Break from writing
1030	Apple	1	To talk with wife
1330	Lentil soup (Progresso)	Bowl	Lunch—this is a high-salt soup
1815	Hamburger on roll	About ¼ lb.	Kim wanted hamburgers and I wanted a salad. Testing light ice cream for dessert.
	Salad with blue cheese	2 Tbs.	
	Light ice cream	2 scoops	
	Tea	1 cup	
2100	Apple	1	Wife & I just talking Sliced apple slowly

Critique: Food was not excessive in calories, but was excessive in sodium (both the hamburger roll and the lentil soup). Everything else was excellent. Since I exercised, I think the food was no problem. I feel great. BP 105/70, Pulse 52 at 8:30 P.M.

Getting in Touch with Yourself

Succeeding at anything requires keeping score. It doesn't follow that you're involved in intense competition; it only means that you need some quantitative scale to chart progress. The simplest health index most people use is climbing on the bathroom scale to chart weight loss, or measuring their waist. In school, progress is a report card; for the athlete it's a time or a score. If you want to get your blood pressure into line, you've got to keep track of your progress. It all has to do with that all-important pump, your heart!

Start with Your Pulse

Measuring your pulse is easy. The doctor usually does it at the wrist, but it can be done in many places. I recommend the wrist because you'll need to use your arm to measure blood pressure and you might as well get accustomed to it right away. You'll need a watch or clock with a second hand; don't use a stop watch.

Place your arm on a table or desk so your elbow is about as high as your heart—that's mid-chest.

Now find your pulse at your wrist. If you're right-handed, use your left hand on your right wrist, pressing with the first two or three fingers on the right side of your right wrist with the palm up. Keep trying until you find the steady beat . . . beat . . . beat. When you can feel it consistently, time it. I prefer that you time it for a full minute. When you get good you can time it for ten seconds and multiply by six, but I'm old-fashioned and believe in getting a good measurement. Count it for a full minute to be sure.

What's a Good Pulse?

From our previous discussion, we know that the peripheral pressure is the result of both the number of beats per minute and the volume of each surge of blood your heart pumps. This implies that a lower pulse rate when resting is consistent with lower blood pressure. Generally, that's the way it is with most people; however, there are limits. Most people seldom have a pulse rate below about 60 beats per

minute, and generally it should be below 80 beats per
minute, with an average of about 70.

Be Consistent

Variations in your pulse can be caused by many things
such as exercise, eating, drinking, tenseness, and anxiety,
to name a few. But, if you take your pulse and your blood
pressure consistently at the same time, under similar conditions, you can develop your "normal" and start to establish
some objectives. Let's take me as an example.

As I write this, I am 52 years old, it is 10:30 A.M., I
exercised vigorously for 30 minutes at 7:00 A.M., ate a
breakfast of melon, oatmeal, and tea at 7:45, read the
paper, and came back to writing at 8:30. So, I'm rested,
relaxed, and working. My pulse is 51 beats per minute. Just
one minute though, I'm an unusual person. I'm in excellent
physical condition for my age, not overweight, and have
healthy parents, and grandparents who were still healthy
into their 80s and 90s.

My wife is another example. She's somewhat over 50,
and her exercise consists of housework and some garden-
ing. She's not athletic, but she does serve as first mate on
our 47-foot ketch. Her pulse is 80. With the exception of 30
minutes of the vigorous exercise I took, and that she slept
to 7:00 A.M., she did and ate what I did. Her normal pulse
rate has been 80 since I can remember . . . it's her normal.

Can You Reduce Your Pulse Rate?

In most cases, yes! It's done by improving your physical
fitness—that is, by developing an exercise program, getting
your weight into line, and improving your diet. Just as
jogging improves the muscle tone of your legs, it similarly
improves the tone of the muscles in your cardiovascular
system. Your heart is a muscle and your arteries and arteri-

oles are lined with muscle cells. To improve the fitness of these muscles, they need to be exercised beyond the normal everyday level. As they become more fit, they don't have to work quite as hard to get all that blood moved around; consequently, as fitness improves, your resting pulse and blood pressure usually decline.

Now, I used jogging as an example, but only because it's a common form of exercise. It can be swimming, brisk walking, cycling, rowing, skating, skiing, and other activities, including skill sports like tennis, handball, and so on. Jumping to conclusions doesn't count! I'll return to exercise in a later chapter, but for now, see it as the means to improve cardiovascular fitness as well as muscle tone.

One word of caution, if you're starting an exercise program for the first time, start slowly. Discuss your plans with your doctor to be sure that the program you select is ambitious enough to be effective and not so ambitious as to be dangerous for you. If you're out of shape, you didn't get that way in a day or two; so, to get into shape, you'll require more than a day or two, in fact, it will require a month or two.

Measure Your Own Blood Pressure

Measuring blood pressure by yourself has become convenient. You can do it in some stores. You can purchase a device like your doctor uses or one of the new electronic, usually battery-operated, devices that are sold in drug stores and other outlets.

The device for measuring blood pressure is called a sphygmomanometer. Big word. Measuring blood pressure is simple. You wrap a band (the cuff) around your arm and stop all blood flow. Then, just below the band, you listen with another device, a stethoscope, to an artery and slowly release the band. As the blood just starts flowing, it's the left ventricle or the *systolic* pressure coming through (the high number), and as the lower pressure comes through, the beats stop and the second sound is steady. That's the background pressure or the *diastolic* pressure (the low number).

The cuff is put into action by pumping it up. It is hooked to a pressure-sensing device. In the doctor's office, it's usually mercury, but now we see more of the newer electronic devices that are calibrated against a standard column of mercury and are almost as accurate. With the electronic device there's no need for the stethoscope, and the sound-sensing device is often more sensitive and objective than the human ear.

I propose you purchase one of the newer battery-operated sphygmomanometers that will give you your systolic and diastolic blood pressures and pulse rate in one reading. I have listed five companies at the end of this chapter that offer excellent products.

How to Measure Your Own Blood Pressure

Your sphygmomanometer will have directions with it. There are a few commonalities that apply to all of them.

- Wrap the cuff snug but not tight.
- Pump the pressure in the cuff sufficiently to stop blood flow; about 200 to 225 millimeters is enough. When you're back in shape, 150 will be plenty.
- Let the air drain from the cuff slowly and steadily.
- Do not take only one measurement, but use several measurements.
- Always measure with your elbow held resting on a table or desk at about the level of your heart, or mid-chest.

Electronic Sphygmomanometers

The battery-operated devices don't always give consistent measurements when there isn't a few minutes between measurements. This is due to current surges. It can also be the result of low batteries. Be sure the batteries are good and give the instrument a few minutes to "settle down."

Mechanical Devices

You're a purist if you purchase the mechanical type where you need the stethoscope and cuff to read the column of mercury. But once you become adept at the measurement, and use the stethoscope effectively, your results will be the most accurate.

You only need to understand what you are listening for: blood flow at two different pressures. The first one is a beat-beat-beat and the second a steady flow. Keep practicing and you will get it correct. If you have trouble, ask a nurse or your doctor to show you.

Is It Necessary to Measure Your Own Blood Pressure?

In my opinion, you should know as much about your body as necessary to regain and maintain optimum health. If you have high blood pressure, or even if you are on the borderline and intend to do something about it, then you should monitor your progress.

I feel obligated to say once again that the more you know and understand about your body, the greater respect you'll have for it. And the better care you'll take of it. To quote Satchel Paige as an old man . . . "Boy, if I'da known I'd need this body so long, I'da taken better care of it."

It's excellent if you have someone who can take your blood pressure regularly for you; for example, a nurse where you work, or a friend. But, the one measurement at the doctor's office, when you're nervous or even anxious, every six or twelve months, is inadequate. And it seems an incredible inconvenience to go to his office once weekly.

Studies have also shown that when people have the doctor take their blood pressure, it's on the high side. Indeed, I discuss the problem called white coat hypertension in Chapter Seventeen.

How Often?

If you seriously plan to control your blood pressure without drugs, you should measure progress daily, or at least weekly. And you should keep the data you accumulate on yourself in your food diary. It's simple: Keep a food diary and at the end of each day include your pulse rate, systolic and diastolic pressure, and make a note about how you feel. Note whether you're relaxed or not. This will give you a running record of your progress and some insight into how your blood pressure relates to how you feel.

One More Time—Why?

Blood pressure, measured regularly and consistently, is a quantitative picture of how your vascular system is working and the wear and tear it is receiving. It is more quantitative—more precise—than most other measurements such as weight, cholesterol, blood sugar, etc. And the beauty of blood pressure is that you can do it yourself quickly and gain an intimate knowledge into the inner workings of your body.

But there's more. As you make progress in gaining control, you'll begin to see how much you control your own health. You'll realize that small changes in diet, a moderate amount of exercise, a diversion, or a hobby can have a profound influence on your health. And you will realize that you are more in control of your health than you ever thought.

Blood Pressure Devices That Work

Item	Company
Astropulse	Marshall Electronics, Inc. 600 Barclay Boulevard Lincolnshire, IL 60069 800-323-1482
Digitronic	Lumiscope Co. 400 Raritan Center Parkway Edison, NJ 08837 800-221-5746
Healthcheck	Healthcheck Corp. 150 Sandbank Rd. Cheshire, CT 06410 800-643-4444
Norelco	North American Philips Corp. High Ridge Park P.O. Box 10166 Stamford, CT 06904 800-243-7884
Tycos	Tycos 95 Old Shoals Road Arden, NC 28704 704-684-4895

Chapter Four

High Blood Pressure Origins I:
Potassium–Sodium Imbalance

Potassium and Sodium

Blood pressure becomes elevated as a result of many factors, including heredity and excessive alcohol consumption, but there's always one common denominator that causes high blood pressure: excessive salt and an incorrect balance between sodium and potassium. We'd better gain a little more understanding of these two materials.

Potassium and sodium are the two major electrolytes found in our bodies. An electrolyte is a nutrient that helps maintain normal nerve conduction, energy production, cell integrity, and many other functions of the body. Electrolytes, as their name implies, conduct electricity. Table salt, sodium chloride, is the most common source of two electrolytes. When added to water, it dissolves and the sodium and chlorine separate to form the electrolytes sodium and chloride. Pure water does not conduct electricity, but water containing salt does. It does because the sodium and chloride are ions, each containing an electric charge.

In your body, there are actually many other minerals, all of which can be called electrolytes, but the three major electrolytes are sodium, potassium, and chloride ions. Other body electrolytes are magnesium, calcium, zinc, and many others in very small amounts. Sodium, potassium, and chlo-

46

ride ions are the electrolytes of greatest abundance and of concern to us. Calcium and magnesium are important as nutrients and, to a lesser extent, as electrolytes.

There are about 50 trillion cells in a human body. These cells are arranged into all the organs and tissues that form a human being: in short, you. Each cell is bathed in fluid, and the inside of each cell is similarly fluid. The fluid both inside and outside the cell contains many materials; most important among them are sodium, potassium, calcium, magnesium, and chloride. The intracellular fluid contains more potassium than sodium, so potassium is the predominant electrolyte inside the cell. The fluid bathing the cell, the extracellular fluid, contains more sodium than potassium, so sodium is the predominant electrolyte in the extracellular fluid. Put another way, there is more potassium inside the cell than outside. Both electrolytes are complemented by chloride. Calcium and magnesium are similar to sodium, more outside than inside. But for now, sodium and potassium are most important.

Shortage of either sodium or potassium is generally not the issue here. We can get plenty of these nutrients from food. In fact, as the story unfolds, you will agree that we get too much sodium.

Balance Is Critical

Having more potassium inside the cell and more sodium outside the cell is important. It enables the cell to carry out all its functions. For example, cells that line the stomach must produce acid and digestive enzymes to break food down. The production of these essential factors requires energy. And if the cells didn't have the correct balance between sodium on the outside and potassium on the inside, it wouldn't work. A second example is nerve impulse conduction. You see how quickly nerve impulses travel if you touch your finger to a hot stove. But more critical is the nerve impulse that tells our hearts to beat. Again, for all these signals to travel properly requires the right ratio of sodium and potassium inside and outside the cell. As a matter of fact, inadequate dietary potassium, often resulting from drastic diets, has been implicated many times in heart attacks.

If I've overdone the point, I'm glad. The ratio of potassium to sodium in our body is very important. And when the ratio becomes seriously distorted, it can be so critical as to be life threatening. Logic dictates that maintaining the correct ratio of potassium to sodium is essential. And when that ratio goes awry, things go wrong.

Three: The Magic Ratio

Your body maintains a ratio of about three parts potassium to one part sodium. This ratio facilitates all the many functions that each cell of each organ and tissue must perform. Indeed, the ratio is not unique to humans and is quite ubiquitous throughout the animal kingdom. In contrast, a much higher ratio is found in the vegetable kingdom. The ratio of potassium to sodium in plants is very high, often over 20 or more. This is because plants don't have, among other things, a nervous system and the need to transmit nerve impulses. This characteristic of plants is to our benefit.

You probably noted that I said the ratio should be "about 3." This implies that it is not precise; well, it isn't. If anything, the ratio could be a little greater than 3. But, for all practical purposes, 3 is the critical ratio.

The book entitled *The K Factor*, which I mentioned in Chapter Two, discusses this ratio in much more depth. In fact, medical scientists are recognizing more and more that a dietary K Factor of 3 or more is essential to optimum health. The problem of too much dietary sodium cannot be overstated. Many people are sensitive to the total amount of salt (sodium chloride) in addition to the K Factor. Therefore, in addition to maintaining a K Factor of 3 or more, the amount of dietary sodium should be maintained below 500 milligrams daily. This translates to about 1,200 milligrams of salt. To be safe, I recommend 1,000 milligrams daily as the absolute upper limit of salt for hypertensives; less is better because most natural foods contain sodium.

Excrete Sodium

Suppose the extracellular fluid, the blood, became oversupplied with sodium. How would the body return things to normal?

The first thing the body would do is excrete more sodium. It does this with the kidneys, the organs that produce urine. But suppose the kidneys don't extract and excrete sufficient sodium from the blood. Well, that becomes a secondary problem that the body is equipped to deal with. Another system cuts in that causes the peripheral vascular system to constrict. Chapter Two teaches that increased resistance to blood flow causes the blood pressure to increase. In this case, increased blood pressure causes the kidneys to excrete more sodium, and when things get right, it returns to normal . . . usually. Elevation of blood pressure to eliminate more sodium shouldn't surprise anyone with engineering knowledge. Man does it all the time with a process called reverse osmosis. In reverse osmosis we simply elevate the pressure to force impurities across a membrane. Unfortunately, when our body must use this process, it's not good.

Dilute Sodium

While the peripheral vascular system is constricted, the body also retains more fluid volume. This extra fluid actually dilutes the extracellular sodium. Look at it this way. While the ratio of sodium to potassium is critical, each individual cell is faced with a concentration of sodium in the external fluid; that is, so much sodium per volume of fluid. Then, the ratio on the basis of cell volume to fluid volume is reduced. A simple device would be for the body to increase its fluid volume; in other words, retain water and thus dilute sodium, making the ratio seem lower. Thus, fluid retention is a phenomenon associated with excess sodium. It enables the kidney to excrete both water and sodium. The only problem is that the blood pressure is elevated to accomplish the task.

Either way, and normally the two mechanisms work together, blood pressure is elevated to eliminate the excess sodium. It's the body's way of returning the potassium–sodium ratio to normal. The only problem is that if this elevation takes place often enough, the blood volume increases and the vascular system adapts and keeps the blood pressure elevated, and normal blood pressure slowly increases until high blood pressure is the outcome.

Diuretics: A Digression

One of the first medical approaches to high blood pressure was to use diuretics. A diuretic causes you to excrete more fluid and with the fluid, sodium chloride—salt. This method usually reduces blood pressure. One major problem with diuretics is that they also cause the kidneys to excrete potassium. This is not good and can cause problems. Along with diuretics, doctors often prescribe potassium supplements as well. The person taking them must also drink more water. Most people who can correct their high blood pressure with diuretics can solve their problems easily with diet.

Dietary Potassium and Sodium: Are We What We Eat?

High blood pressure results from excessive sodium and the need to maintain a correct potassium–sodium balance in the body. Unequivocally, diet has a profound effect.

From our simple discussion of excess sodium, you know that excess sodium comes from the food we eat; similarly, inadequate potassium is primarily the result of diet. After all, both these electrolytes come from the food we eat and beverages we drink.

Initially, based on Dahl's famous studies, scientists thought excessive dietary sodium was the culprit. Then around 1974, some papers started appearing in medical journals that indicated potassium intake was also important. Epidemiologists, medical detectives, found that when the dietary potassium to sodium ratio—the K factor—falls below 3 to about 1 or even 1.5, high blood pressure increases dramatically. Research on ethnic groups that have more high blood pressure and diabetic children (who are especially likely to get high blood pressure) leaves no doubt that the dietary potassium–sodium ratio is critical. This finding, indeed this breakthrough in our knowledge, throws the responsibility back on the individual; after all, you control the food you eat.

Other, less direct support comes from observing nature. If you examine natural foods for potassium and sodium, you will quickly see that they invariably contain much more potassium than sodium. Indeed, the ratio in animal foods of 3 is low compared to vegetables where the ratio is often 10 or more. Natural foods simply contain much more potassium than sodium. In fact, estimates by some anthropologists place the potassium to sodium ratio in the diet of our remote ancestors of 10,000 years ago at about 16! Now, that figure is really high and is debatable. But suppose it's high by 50%; that still puts the ratio at 8. Man's natural diet was once much higher in potassium than in sodium. The margin is not close. So, if we lived in harmony with nature, our K Factor would be 3 or more.

As a preview of things to come later, I'll tell you now that the average diet today—that probably includes yours—contains more sodium than potassium. That means the body must literally work overtime to excrete the excess sodium and retain potassium. And, from the preceding discussion, you see that one way the body accomplishes this task is to raise blood pressure. So, we are what we eat; if we eat for high blood pressure, eventually we'll get it.

How Much Potassium and Sodium Do We Need?

Although the ratio of potassium to sodium is probably more important than the absolute amount of either, there does appear to be a minimum of about 200 or 250 milligrams daily of sodium required by the average adult. That translates to 650 milligrams of salt. And the requirement for potassium is about 1,000 milligrams. Those numbers are not minimums; they are the levels to maintain good health. They tell an important story; we require a lot more potassium than sodium. Indeed, the Food and Nutrition Board describes a safe and adequate range as 1,100 to 3,300 milligrams of sodium and 1,875 to 5,625 milligrams of potassium.

Safe and adequate does not mean "required." It means that most people can consume sodium in that range and remain in satisfactory health. But, to the government satisfactory health means "free from overt symptoms," and their numbers were established before we understood the K Factor.

I suggest the government rewrite its recommendations, proposing an upper limit of about 1,500 milligrams of sodium and a ratio of potassium to sodium, a K Factor, of at least 3. And for people whose diastolic blood pressure has reached 85, their sodium limit should be reduced to 1,000 milligrams with a K Factor of 4 or more. No matter what numbers you use, the K Factor should be at least 3. When I look at the abundance of nature and examine its fundamentals, I conclude that the dietary K Factor should probably be even greater than 4, perhaps as high as 10.

Evidence? It's in the Urine

There's a great deal of scientific evidence to support the notion of more dietary potassium than sodium. It comes from an examination of people's urine.

Remember the need to restore the potassium–sodium ratio that elevates blood pressure in the first place. If the ratio is correct, there's no need for the body to compensate by elevating blood pressure. So, why not look at the ratio of these electrolytes in the urine and see if there's a correlation? When medical scientists do just that, they find that there is a clear trend. If a person's ratio is 3 or higher, high blood pressure is almost nonexistent. As it approaches a ratio of 1, blood pressure increases dramatically. In fact, if these ratios are the averages for a group, the number of people with high blood pressure jumps from just 1% or 2% to over 20%. There is simply no doubt about the need to maintain a potassium–sodium ratio of 3 or more.

Dietary Changes to Make Now

As I lay the groundwork for your new dietary plan, one important part should be obvious: Increase the potassium and decrease the sodium in your diet. Actually, nature will do this for you if you'll just give her a reasonable chance. Natural foods, especially vegetable foods, are naturally high in potassium and low in sodium. In contrast, many man-made and highly processed foods are exactly the opposite: high in sodium and low in potassium. Therefore, most of these changes should be obvious.

1. Eat one to three fresh vegetables of any type at every meal except breakfast. These include salads, grains, tubers (e.g., potatoes), beans (except black beans), cereals, peas, and many other vegetables you can think of. Always boil, steam, or stir fry. Never add salt.

2. Start each day with a cereal that has more potassium than sodium. Some examples include oatmeal made without salt, Nabisco Shredded Wheat, Bran Buds, puffed rice, wheat germ, and Quaker 100% Natural. Always use low-fat or skim milk.
3. Don't eat any processed food product that doesn't clearly have the potassium and sodium content declared on the label. And the potassium must be at least two times the sodium!
4. No processed meat products at all! This includes sausages of all kinds and processed poultry.
5. Do not use salt on any foods. This will be tough, but you can do it. Alternatives are to use a hot pepper sauce such as Tabasco, horseradish, or salt substitutes. Herbs, spices, onions, and garlic go well with meat.
6. For dessert, learn to use fresh fruit whenever possible. You can also eat ice cream, ice milk, and sherbet. You must not eat baked goods, pies or cakes.
7. Purchase one of the low-sodium cookbooks listed in Chapter Fourteen.

While some of these changes might be contrary to the way you have been eating, taken together, they are a first, giant step toward reducing your blood pressure. More than that, once they become habit, you will be on your way to optimizing your health.

Chapter Five

High Blood Pressure Origins II: Overweight and Fitness

Is It Mechanical?

One sure way to reduce blood pressure in most people is for them to lose weight. As the excess weight comes off, the blood pressure declines—and it usually declines more rapidly than the weight loss. Every study on blood pressure shows that the more overweight people are, the more likely they are to have high blood pressure. If the same people simply reduce, their blood pressure declines. But surprisingly, we are not completely sure how overweight produces high blood pressure.

Intuitively, we can see that carrying excess pounds causes the heart to work harder. For example, if you're 15 pounds overweight, whenever you climb the stairs your heart must work harder; it doesn't matter that it's 15 pounds of fat and not a box of books. The same extra work is required. But 15 pounds of fat are worse than 15 pounds of books because each pound of fat requires about 5 miles of extra blood capillaries. The increased blood flow required by all the extra capillaries requires harder and more rapid pumping by the heart, and that usually translates to higher blood pressure.

Undoubtedly, this mechanical explanation accounts for much of the high blood pressure we see in overweight people. Indeed, I have conducted studies in which over-weight people with high blood pressure are put on reducing diets. It's rewarding to observe how gratified they are as the blood pressure comes down with the weight loss. And to see how much better they feel about themselves because they look better. They gain a new lease on life. The excessive weight–high blood pressure relationship goes beyond the mechanical requirement for more pumping action, however. It's more complex and involves metabolism.

Is It Insulin?

When we put overweight people on a low-calorie diet with a potassium–sodium ratio of 3 or more, their blood pressure starts to decline within five days or less, even before there's much weight loss. By the time they've lost about a third of their excess weight, their blood pressure is usually normal. While these results leave little doubt that overweight produces high blood pressure, they also indicate that something else is at work. Most medical researchers believe that the extra factor is the hormone insulin.

I saw this phenomenon at work in a man whose case describes it quite clearly.

Ralph's Story

Ralph is 45, overweight, and has high blood pressure. He is on medication and dislikes taking it. All he needs to do is lose weight—about 25 pounds, but he likes to experiment with himself and because he has a theory about toxins, he goes on a self-imposed water and juice fast to eliminate. On this fast, he simply drinks water and grapefruit juice for a week. In his words: "Within 24 hours of following the water diet, my blood pressure is back to normal and I lose a few pounds. I drink only unsweetened grapefruit juice and water for a week and I feel great. I lose about 10 pounds in that time and everything is normal. It takes about three days for the toxins to leave. I just can't follow a diet like that full time."

Ralph's story is an excellent account of the role insulin plays in high blood pressure. The only "toxin" involved is salt! By not putting any more salt into his body, restoring a good K Factor, and reducing his calories and sugar intake to almost nothing, Ralph simply eliminates his need for any insulin output and allows his body to flush out the salt. Insulin causes the body to retain salt. With the minor amount of sugar from unsweetened grapefruit juice, his body doesn't need to produce any insulin. Then, as his body eliminates its salt (call it Ralph's toxin), it releases the fluid it retained because of the salt, and two things happen. Ralph's blood pressure drops—no more extra fluid—and since water weighs eight pounds per gallon, he drops about eight pounds of water. Since he didn't eat, he probably loses another pound or two of fat.

Ralph's is an excellent account of how to delude yourself into a belief in something mysterious and unexplainable, in his case, "toxins." His account shows that fluid retention in hypertensives is serious and that they lose weight and blood pressure quickly as a result. Let me explain.

How Insulin Works

Your body secretes the hormone insulin so it can metabolize the simple sugar, glucose, that circulates in your blood. When you eat, your blood sugar level rises as you absorb sugar and other nutrients from your food, and specialized cells in your pancreas produce insulin to facilitate metabolism of the blood glucose. As it is metabolized, or stored as glycogen, blood sugar is returned to its normal level. But overweight people often have flaws in insulin utilization. The extra fat cells require a higher level of insulin production. This is not simply the outcome of having more cells, but it involves the ability or inability of these cells to use the insulin. The net outcome is that the body produces more insulin to compensate.

If insulin only dealt with glucose metabolism, there would be no problem, but insulin does more. A secondary function of insulin is to help the kidneys retain sodium. In short, the excess insulin results in less sodium excretion. From the discussion in Chapter Four, you know that this results in greater fluid retention. Fluid retention results in higher blood pressure.

Another way to visualize what happens here is to look at it this way. By retaining sodium, the kidneys put the body on a "high-sodium" diet even though you might not be eating excess sodium. This causes the body to increase fluid and indirectly reduce the level of blood sugar. Don't forget: Elevated blood sugar is not good; in fact, it's a disease called diabetes. So, in summary, the body is actually protecting itself against one evil, elevated blood sugar, by creating a lesser evil, high blood pressure.

Back to Ralph

When Ralph goes on his fluid fast, he relieves his body of the need to produce extra insulin. There's simply no food intake, so he doesn't elevate blood glucose. The lack of extra insulin permits his kidneys to excrete sodium normally. As the sodium goes, the excess fluid is excreted, the blood pressure declines, and Ralph is happy because he loses weight, his blood pressure returns to normal, and for a few days he feels great. He's normal again. But, it doesn't last. In Ralph's own words: "As soon as I go back to eating, even if I don't eat much, the weight increases and the blood pressure with it. In a couple of weeks, I'm back on medication."

As soon as Ralph starts consuming food again, carbohydrates enter his blood as glucose. This triggers the normal production of insulin, but Ralph's excess weight makes him less sensitive to insulin, so his body produces more. The slight excess causes his kidneys to retain sodium. The extra sodium retention causes more fluid retention and the weight comes back very quickly.

But Ralph never needs to return to blood pressure medication. What Ralph needs to do is lose weight on a good diet balanced in potassium and sodium so he'll never need the medication again.

Carbohydrate

Chapter Ten explains the difference between simple and complex carbohydrates. The objective is to obtain your simple carbohydrates from fruits and vegetables and the bulk of your carbohydrates as starches from vegetables, grains, and cereals. Let me describe an experiment that makes my point. Apples contain carbohydrate in three forms: simple sugars, glucose and fructose; complex carbohydrates as starch; carbohydrate as dietary fiber. In the experiment, conducted in England, people were given either a whole apple, or an apple that had been pureed, removing the fiber and starches. Blood sugars and insulin levels were compared when people got the same amount of carbohydrate as the apple or as the totally pureed and completely clarified juice.

You've probably guessed that the apple caused the least insulin response and the clarified juice caused the greatest insulin release. The reason is basic. Natural foods provide carbohydrate in a matrix that contains simple sugars, natural starches, and nondigestible carbohydrates called fiber. Taken together, these factors modulate the absorption of the simple sugars, glucose and fructose, and reduce the output of insulin.

It's a good practice for everyone to follow the dietary changes I've described. But it's especially important for people who tend to be overweight, and anyone who has even slightly elevated blood pressure.

The Spa Rip-off

Several years ago, I was commissioned to go to Europe and evaluate mineral spas. These places, usually located at natural mineral springs, cater to people who make an annual or semi-annual visit, usually for a week, to "take the cure." The cure usually consists of at least three or four long daily walks to drink the water directly from the spring. Additionally, bottles of spring water are available everywhere in the spa.

Participants are put on a natural-food, low-calorie diet with no alcohol. In addition, if they are too overweight to exercise vigorously, the long walks to the spring are usually much more exercise than they get normally. There's usually an additional walking program. Does it surprise you that, in addition to shedding a few pounds, their high blood pressure is dramatically reduced, albeit temporarily? It's just a different version of Ralph's story.

Low calories, reduced insulin production, balanced potassium–sodium, and some exercise. It all adds up to allowing the body to function normally. The body is able to reduce its insulin output, excrete excess sodium and the retained fluid it causes. Everyone is happy, especially the spa proprietor.

Do All Overweight People Get High Blood Pressure?

It is the exceptions that lead medical scientists to understand the marvelous workings of the human body. There are many overweight people who do not develop high blood pressure until they get older. And that has led scientists to understand better the influence of insulin on sodium retention.

Some people can tolerate extra fat without excessive insulin production. And some people have kidneys that are not as sensitive to extra insulin. Therefore, they do not retain sodium and their blood pressure remains normal. While these overweight people still have the burden of extra weight, and their hearts must work harder, their hearts produce sufficient blood flow without having to produce higher pressure. We say that they simply have a "high stroke volume," meaning that with each pump of the heart, more blood is expelled.

Time eventually works against these exceptional people, however, and as they get older, their blood pressure begins to creep higher. And often, within a short time, less than a year, their blood pressure will go from normal to high. They are then faced with a long period of serious dieting or a life that will include daily medication.

Putting It All Together: A Clinical Study

With several researchers at the Scripps Clinic, I conducted a clinical study with a large group of people who were overweight and had high blood pressure. They were divided into two groups and put on an 800-calorie, well balanced liquid formula diet. Since the diet had been thoroughly tested, there was no doubt that each group would lose weight at approximately the same rate. But we also changed the potassium–sodium ratio.

The liquid formula was adjusted in one group, call it the blue group, so they had a K Factor of a little less than 1. The other group, call it the gold group, got the standard liquid formula with its K Factor of 3. You should be able to predict the outcome. Both groups lost weight at about the same rate, although the gold group lost weight a little more quickly. The big difference was in blood pressure.

Blood pressure in the gold group came down very quickly. In fact, in the first week, many of them returned to normal. Not so with the blue group. Even though they lost weight, the imbalance of potassium and sodium made their bodies retain more fluid and maintain a higher blood pressure. As the study moved into its fourth week, even the blue group was getting normal blood pressure readings and they lost more weight. This study proves several points about blood pressure in overweight people.

Let's Review Overweight Again

Significant weight loss causes overweight people to regain normal blood pressure. This effect is somewhat mechanical—the heart has less work to do—because fluid loss and fat loss require the heart to pump less blood through less tissue.

- A diet of complex carbohydrates from natural food accelerates blood pressure reduction due to reduced insulin output.
- A diet balanced with a K Factor of 3 or more requires less fluid retention, and blood pressure returns to normal more quickly.
- Normal blood pressure continues if the person maintains the new weight. This requires a diet balanced in potassium, sodium, and complex carbohydrates, low in sugar consumption, and not excessive in calories.

Fitness: The Counterpart of Overweight

A radio talk show interviewer once asked me to describe my fitness program. When I told him how I've maintained an aerobic program for over 20 years, he gasped.

"Dr. Scala, when the urge to exercise strikes me, I immediately lie down until the urge goes away."

I thought, "Where have I heard that before?" as I watched my host light up a cigarette.

Please, get one thing straight. An exercise program doesn't mean you have to jog two or more miles daily. Indeed, it simply means regular, moderate exercise such as vigorous walking for a period of 30 minutes three or four times each week. More vigorous exercise can be done for 20 minutes but also three or four times weekly.

People Are Sedentary

At a recent symposium for older adults, I gave some statistics that made the audience gasp. Americans own more jogging shoes than any other population. Over 90% of jogging shoe owners don't put them on more than once each week!

Many American corporations make exercise facilities available to employees. These range from a jogging track with showers available, to elaborate indoor facilities staffed by experts. Most supply exercise apparel with free laundry service. The employee supplies the shoes, energy, and time. I was asked to speak on the subject at a major corporation, so I did a survey to get a feeling of how extensively these facilities are used. I defined regular use as three times weekly for 45 minutes or more. By this definition, the employees use the facilities to the whopping level of 3% in most companies, as high as 5% in others.

So, when you see joggers in the parks and on the roads, don't conclude that "everyone is doing it." You are seeing the small percentage who does and not the other 95% to 97% that "lies down until the urge passes."

Does Fitness Affect Blood Pressure?

In general, people who maintain a minimal level of fitness have lower blood pressure over their entire lifetime. Many studies have been conducted where hypertensives begin an exercise program with or without a weight-loss program, and the results are always the same—the blood pressure declines. There simply isn't any doubt or debate any longer: Cardiovascular fitness is an important part of blood pressure management.

How Does It Work?

Regular vigorous exercise helps to reduce blood pressure. Since exercise generates metabolic heat, that heat must be dissipated by radiating into the atmosphere if running and into water if swimming. The body accomplishes this task by increasing the peripheral blood flow and removing heat by evaporating sweat. You can sweat while swimming.

During exercise, blood pressure will increase somewhat because the heart pumps faster to get the blood flowing more rapidly to both nourish the muscles and dissipate the heat. But, after exercise is finished, the relaxed muscles and dilated peripheral capillaries allow the blood to flow more freely and the blood pressure declines.

A second important influence of exercise has to do with insulin. There's no longer any doubt that a fit individual manages insulin more effectively. This includes diabetics who must use insulin injections twice daily and adult onset diabetics who usually get that way by being overweight. It also includes people like me who don't have diabetes or high blood pressure.

Exercise helps to reduce the circulating levels of insulin. The level of insulin influences the reabsorption of sodium by the kidneys that are discussed in Chapter Eight. It's all interrelated. Reduced insulin helps to reduce the blood pressure indirectly by influencing the kidneys to reabsorb less sodium. This is discussed in Chapter Eight and illustrates the relationship between diet and lifestyle.

Jean's Story

Jean is a beautiful woman of 33. She's always had a weight problem, and mild hypertension has appeared in the last three years. Her physician put her on the first level of medication, a diuretic. Since I was conducting a program for people with high blood pressure, she volunteered. In this study the participants received capsules of either a placebo or an active substance that helped to reduce blood pressure, and they were asked to participate in a supervised aerobic exercise and diet program. This exercise consisted of a vigorous walking program and 30 minutes of aerobic exercise daily. The exercise was vigorous, but coordinated with the fitness of the participants so they didn't become too stiff. Jean received a placebo for part of the study and the active substance for the other. The results indicated that with regular exercise, she was fine and didn't need the medication. I received the following note from her about two months after she started.

> Dear Dr. Scala:
> I just returned from my doctor. She told me I can go without medication as long as I keep up my exercise program and my weight down. I can't tell you how thankful I am for your interest. I feel like my whole life has changed. I'm still losing weight and plan to keep up the diet plan you gave me.

The letter continues, but the point is clear. Exercise helps; it helped Jean. She did better when she exercised and dieted. The substance being tested didn't work for Jean, but exercise and weight loss did. She's proof.

A Clinical Study: What's Fitness?

A study was conducted at the famous Aerobic Institute in Dallas, Texas, to evaluate the effects of weight loss and exercise on total cardiovascular fitness and body tone. In every case, the best program included diet and exercise. Although dieters increase cardiovascular fitness just by losing weight, it's more effective if they exercise as well.

Similarly, if exercisers diet for either weight loss or simply to improve health, as well as exercise, they gain more cardiovascular fitness than if they only exercise. This indicates that fitness, good weight, and other lifestyle habits are all part of "fitness."

Correct exercise causes your heart to beat faster while you're doing it, and it should last for 20 to 45 minutes depending on its intensity. First, your doctor is the best judge of how vigorous exercise can be for you. For example, is it safe for you to jog at 8 minutes a mile, or should you stick to walking? Is swimming okay, a stationary bike, or a simulated cross-country ski device like the one I use?

Generally speaking, if your heart is sound and you're not seriously overweight, walking or slow jogging is fine. That means the exercise devices (bike, etc.) will work for you as well. So the question is, how long?

Exercise doesn't do any good until it's done for at least 10 minutes, and if it's not done vigorously (e.g., walking), it should last for 45 minutes; a slow jog should last about 25 to 30 minutes. I strongly urge you to purchase *The Aerobics Program for Total Well Being* by Kenneth Cooper. This both will help you precisely determine your fitness level and plan your exercise needs with similar precision. By exercising effectively, you can restore your fitness to its optimum level.

How Old?

Don't worry about being too old. My mother is 82 and she uses her stationary bicycle 15 to 20 minutes daily. She has arthritis in her knees and walking is hard on her and dangerous where she lives; hence, the bike. Similarly, a 94-year-old man came to hear me speak once. After my talk, he told me how he walks 40 minutes daily, rain or shine.

You're never too old!

Chapter Six

High Blood Pressure Origins III:
Calcium, Magnesium, and Alcohol

Essential Minerals

Calcium and magnesium are minerals that are essential for health. Calcium is the mineral that is the basis of strong bones and teeth, but it is also required for muscle function, nerve function, and more. Therefore, getting sufficient calcium either from foods or food supplements is essential. We require at least 800 milligrams of calcium daily and there is a rapidly growing consensus among health researchers that we need more. Some people, especially women, need as much as 1,500 milligrams daily. That's why we call it a macromineral, because 800 milligrams is a lot. Dietary surveys indicate that less than 40% of us get the 800 milligrams daily from our diet, let alone 1,500 milligrams. Milk and other dairy products are the major source of calcium. In fact, 800 milligrams of calcium is the equivalent of about 3 glasses of milk daily and 1,500 milligrams is about 5 glasses. The equivalent in cheese would be unacceptable on this plan so the only alternative is deep green vegetables such as spinach and broccoli. But 800 milligrams of calcium requires about 8 stalks of broccoli or about 25 ounces of spinach; both unlikely amounts to be eaten. Indeed, most dietary surveys indicate that Americans don't consume nearly enough milk or deep green vegetables to obtain the 800

67

milligrams, let alone the consensus panel's 1,500 milligrams. And since calcium is so essential to good health, calcium supplements make good sense. In many cases, they are the only recourse.

In later chapters we'll come back to these discussions about what we get and don't get from food. But at this time, please recognize that you probably don't get sufficient calcium or magnesium from your diet. And, I strongly urge you to think of using more milk in your diet, or supplements that supply both calcium and magnesium. An excellent research study recently published in *The Journal of Clinical Nutrition* shows once and for all that your body uses calcium and magnesium from supplements as well as from food.

Just as the ratio of potassium and sodium is important to each living cell, so is the ratio of calcium outside the cell to calcium inside the cell. This is because calcium is an essential element required by the cell membrane to maintain its integrity. If the ratio of calcium outside the cell to calcium inside the cell drops, as it can if we either don't get enough enough calcium or we excrete too much, the cell membrane loses it integrity, becomes "leaky," and allows sodium to enter and potassium to leak out, and along with that lets more calcium in!

When calcium levels inside the muscle cell become too high, the cell becomes tense; it tightens up. You might ask, "So what?" So tighter peripheral muscles that line the arterioles means the arterioles and capillaries are more constricted. Now, recall that blood pressure increases as peripheral resistance to blood flow increases (that's the flow of blood in the muscles, the skin, and the surface of the body in general). In short, the heart has to pump harder to force the blood through the myriad of capillaries involved.

Therefore, calcium is necessary for more blood pressure, and when it is in inadequate supply it can cause the blood pressure to rise. This effect of calcium is what we call "indirect," because it's not primary to high blood pressure. But, each of these effects add up to a problem, and effective dietary control doesn't leave one stone unturned. Another negative in the calcium story is that recent research indicates that excess sodium seems to cause more calcium excretion. So, not only are our diets usually inadequate in calcium, but that aspect is made worse by excessive sodium.

The Old Garden Hose Analogy

Water flows smoothly through a garden hose until you either fold it over to stop the flow completely, or fold it a little to slow the flow down, or constrict it with some kind of clamping device. And as you do any one of these, the pressure in the hose between the constriction and the faucet increases. In fact, you can even see the hose become swollen, and leaks sometimes spring at weak points.

The garden hose analogy is very good because it helps us visualize what happens when peripheral resistance increases. Tiny muscles surrounding the arterioles tighten down and constrict them. Constricted arterioles produce restricted blood flow. Restricted blood flow, like the constricted garden hose, means higher blood pressure between the heart and the surface. And, without getting ahead of the story, the leaks in the hose have their counterparts in blood vessels. The only difference is the damaged item is not easily replaced at the hardware store.

Magnesium

Magnesium is another mineral that is essential to many bodily functions. It is required for muscle contraction and many processes in metabolism. Nutritionists classify it with calcium as a macromineral, because we require 400 milligrams daily. Most of our magnesium comes from milk, meat, and vegetables. But, since milk is the major source, dietary surveys indicate that only about 50% of people get the correct amount of magnesium daily.

This dietary shortfall results from dairy products, especially milk, vegetables and water systems lacking in magnesium. In my opinion, nutritionists, dieticians, and doctors don't give magnesium its due. So the public remains generally uniformed.

Magnesium, like calcium, is necessary for membrane integrity—and integrity of the membrane is essential for the maintenance of the correct potassium–sodium–calcium ratio. Ultimately, this membrane integrity influences peripheral resistance, because it will cause the muscles to either relax or to remain tense.

Since low blood levels of magnesium have been associated with high blood pressure, a reason other than its membrane effects on the potassium–sodium–calcium system has been sought. There is some evidence to show that a hormone, renin (Chapters Two and Eight), is elevated when blood levels of magnesium are reduced. Since elevated renin produces elevated blood pressure, the connection is obvious.

How Much Calcium? Magnesium?

Unfortunately, I can't say that a precise level of dietary calcium will prevent high blood pressure from occurring. That is because potassium, sodium, and magnesium are all involved. In nutrition, nothing stands alone; teamwork is important.

I can make a promise. As you restore the natural potassium–sodium ratio, you will need only the recommended daily allowance of about 800 milligrams of calcium and 400 milligrams of magnesium. If you are a woman before menopause, 1,000 milligrams of calcium is appropriate, and for postmenopausal woman, 1,500 milligrams is better.

Salt

Although high blood pressure is mostly about potassium and sodium, it's also about table salt. Table salt is sodium chloride; by weight it's about 40% sodium and 60% chloride. In natural foods, even those high in sodium, it's not often found as sodium chloride. Indeed, it's found as sodium bicarbonate or the sodium salt of organic acids such as sodium citrate.

When these other sodium salts are used in experiments on high blood pressure, they don't have the same elevating effect as sodium chloride, common table salt. The reason for this relates to how the kidneys function and the presence of chloride around the cell membrane.

The kidney requires chloride for sodium reabsorption and sodium for chloride reabsorption. It's no doubletalk; it means that the kidney reabsorbs salt from the urine it is producing. Some other evidence suggests that in the peripheral cells, chloride facilitates the transport of sodium into each cell. This is more evidence that the major culprit in high blood pressure is sodium chloride, common salt, and not only sodium.

Sodium (Salt) Sensitivity

The bottom line of all this is the identification of table salt, or sodium chloride, as a culprit.

For many years we spoke of "sodium-sensitive" hypertensives; now we speak of them as "salt-sensitive" hypertensives. These are normal-weight people with high blood pressure who are very responsive to salt. Reduce their salt intake to 1,000 milligrams or less daily and their high blood pressure seems to disappear. I should add that a person consuming 1,000 milligrams or less salt daily is on a pretty natural diet, so his or her K Factor would be 5 or more. By making one change this person will have controlled three important variables at the same time: low sodium, low salt, and an excellent K Factor.

People often ask, "Who's salt or sodium sensitive?" Believe me, I wanted to know that too, so I consulted an expert, Dr. Edwin (Eli) Whitney, a brilliant cardiologist who conducts a powerful preventive medicine program at Brooks Medical Center in San Antonio, Texas. He works with people with high blood pressure all the time, so I asked him: "Eli, how many hypertensives would you estimate are salt sensitive?" His answer was clear and to the point.

"Fifty percent!"

A thorough search of the medical literature confirms Dr. Whitney's answer, with one caveat: Some people are more sensitive than others. In other words, some require a sodium-restricted diet of less than 500 milligrams of sodium daily and others can get along with about 800 milligrams. That translates to 1,000 to 1,500 milligrams of salt daily. I recommend, as he does, the 1,000-milligram level. A diet emphasizing natural foods will generally supply adequate sodium and remain well within the 1,000-milligram salt limit.

Alcohol

In 1967, the classic Los Angeles Heart Study established a link between alcohol consumption and high blood pressure. As alcohol consumption increases, so does blood pressure. And it has been confirmed in study after study. All these studies show a clear relationship between long-term alcohol consumption and high blood pressure. In fact, the Harvard Medical School Health Letter estimates that alcohol consumption accounts for from 5% to 25% of essential hypertension pressure!

Now, don't get the idea that everyone who has a cocktail in the evening, or a glass of wine at dinner, will develop high blood pressure. That's not the point. It's not the occasional drink; it's regular drinking. But that doesn't mean only heavy drinking is implicated. It appears that about four cans of beer, two or more glasses of wine, or about three drinks with one ounce of liquor on a daily basis is enough to cause high blood pressure in many individuals. Conversely, the same research indicates that the equivalent of one beer daily, or a glass of wine, or one drink will not cause high blood pressure in most people. That suggests that if you drink moderately, you'll have no problem.

Charlie's Story

In one of my lectures I gave the bare bones of what's in this book as the means to reduce blood pressure. I got a letter from Charlie, a man in Colorado, about a month later, that went like this:

Dear Dr. Scala:
I've been following the advice you gave at your lecture in Denver. I've reduced my weight, stopped smoking, and have been taking potassium supplements with no results.

The letter went on to describe that his doctor had prescribed the potassium supplements. Since the doctor's prescription conflicts with what I advise, a call was in order. Boy, did I get a different picture.

Charlie had indeed lost some weight. But he retained all his bad habits. He faithfully drank three to five ounces of Tennessee sipping whiskey each evening. For lunch he had sliced beef with gravy, and his weigh reduction was 10 pounds, from 220 to 210; he should be about 185 for his 5'11" frame. His doctor, being conscientious, applied a little, much too little, logic and felt that if he restored Charlie's potassium–sodium ratio, it would compensate for his poor dietary habits. He didn't quite get the K Factor message. You don't simply add potassium.

I called the doctor and we set up a simple plan: a good weight loss program, no more whiskey, and the dietary rules in this book to restore potassium–sodium balance.

Within a week, Charlie's blood pressure had dropped so his diastolic was below 90. As of this writing, two months later, his weight's down to 195, his blood pressure's still higher than I like, 135/85, but he doesn't require medication. Charlie also learned something that other regular drinkers learn. If he starts the booze again, the blood pressure goes up directly.

High blood pressure from excessive alcohol is not good; the only way to reverse it is to stop drinking. Drugs that usually work for high blood pressure don't usually work for drinkers. So as they say, "get off the sauce," or at least reduce it to the level of one drink daily.

How Does Alcohol Work?

Much is known about how alcohol affects the body, but no one is sure about how it elevates blood pressure. We can speculate on two possible mechanisms, however.

Some specialists believe that it directly influences the hormones that either elevate or reduce blood pressure. It simply throws the system out of balance. The hormones that elevate blood pressure are simply overproduced and the organs don't get the signal to stop. That would explain why alcohol-related high blood pressure is refractory to the usual drugs. It also explains why when the booze stops, the blood pressure returns to normal.

A second explanation is similar to the calcium story. Alcohol simply alters the potassium–sodium–calcium–magnesium balance, the tension of the cells increases, and peripheral resistance increases. This causes constriction of the capillaries with an increase of the peripheral resistance. High blood pressure follows. This explanation also squares with the lack of effectiveness of drugs. And it teaches that when the booze stops, the blood pressure returns to normal. I like this explanation.

What's the Take Away?

If you're like Charlie, stop drinking! It's that simple.

Under any circumstances, if there's even a hint that your elevated blood pressure is alcohol related, *stop!*

If you're truly in control of yourself, reduce your alcohol intake to no more than a glass of wine or one mixed drink daily. And if your blood pressure remains above normal at that level, you should stop altogether.

Remember, alcohol has negative effects on your body besides the high blood pressure. If it's elevating your blood pressure, it's reducing the quality and quantity of your life in many other ways. Only you can do anything about it; and the only thing to do is stop!

Put This Knowledge to Work

Another section of this book gets deeply into the dietary approaches to reduce blood pressure, but I can't wait. You should have gained much insight by this time, but let's establish some specific and practical dos and don'ts right now.

Do eat foods rich in calcium and magnesium. That means milk, yogurt, dark green vegetables, like broccoli and spinach, beans, and potatoes.

Do drink mineral water with low sodium if you live in a water-softened area, or, if you have a water softener in your home, use bottled water for drinking.

Do use a balanced food supplement that contains about 50% of the U.S. RDA of the nutrients. If it doesn't contain sufficient magnesium and calcium, use a separate supplement.

Do use calcium supplements; take up to 600 milligrams of calcium daily.

Don't have more than one drink or glass of beer. Hopefully, you will stop all but an occasional drink or glass of wine.

Don't use table salt at the table or in cooking. Substitute with onions, onion powder, garlic, garlic powder, or a few drops of Tabasco sauce. We'll cover this in detail later.

Chapter Seven

High Blood Pressure Origins IV: Balancing Fat

Soft versus Hard Fat

What do a stick of butter and a bottle of olive oil have in common? They're both fat and provide 9 calories per gram—that's 252 calories per ounce—or about 85 per tablespoon. But the olive oil is much better for you than the butter.

Most animal fat, for example butter or the white fat around beef, is solid at room temperature. In contrast, vegetable fat—more specifically vegetable oil—is liquid at room temperature. It's obvious why nutritionists call animal fat "hard fat" and vegetable oil "soft fat."

Saturated versus Unsaturated

The difference is in the chemical structure of the two fats. Chemists tell us the structure of hard fat is very dense and uniform. Highly saturated is the term used. There's no open space to add anything further. In contrast, the vegetable oils are not dense and uniform. They contain spaces that are open and reactive, so things can be added. Unsaturated is how they are described.

The terms saturated and unsaturated refer specifically to the actual chemical structure called the molecular configuration. In a saturated fat, the actual linkages holding carbon atoms together are all used up; that's why I used the terms dense and uniform. In an unsaturated fat, the linkages holding the carbon atoms together are not all used up; that's why I said there are some open spaces and they are more reactive.

Don't let the chemistry scare you; just get accustomed to the idea that oils are unsaturated and hard fats are saturated.

MFA, PUFA, SFA

Olive oil is an excellent example of an oil that has only one open space. Monounsaturated fatty acid (MFA) is the term used to describe it. While MFA oils are liquid at room temperature, they, like olive oil, tend to be amber in color and somewhat thick. Moderately viscous is the appropriate term.

Sunflower oil is an excellent example of an oil that has many open spaces. Polyunsaturated fatty acid (PUFA) is the term we use to describe these light oils. There can be varying degrees to PUFA. The more unsaturated they are, the lighter in color and the more fluid, less viscous, they are.

Beef lard is an excellent example of saturated fatty acids (SFA). SFA is not liquid at room temperature; in fact, it is white and hard. And this is true of most animal fat. The most common examples are beef and pork fat.

Good News and Bad News

Good news: Polyunsaturated fats help to keep blood pressure normal. In fact, we'll see shortly that some oils, especially vegetable and fish oils, can help reduce blood pressure. Vegetable oil supplies linoleic acid, an oil from plants that is essential for health. Linoleic acid is the raw material for a substance the body produces named prostaglandin number two, PG2 for short. PG2 and other materials produced from it are important in the relaxation and contraction of the muscles that line the arterioles. Therefore, linoleic acid has a metabolic effect that helps to maintain normal blood pressure.

PUFAs also reduce blood pressure by reducing blood viscosity. Remember from Chapter Two that reduced viscosity decreases total peripheral resistance to blood flow. And decreased resistance means lower blood pressure.

Bad news: Saturated fats have a mild tendency to increase blood pressure. The saturated fats have a negative effect by increasing blood viscosity. Increased viscosity contributes to total peripheral resistance, and that increases blood pressure. Obviously, the dietary objective should be to reduce saturated fat and to emphasize the unsaturated fat in the diet. These changes are achieved by shifting emphasis from meat and butter to foods that deliver the unsaturated fats.

Down with Cholesterol: A Digression

There's another reason to eat more PUFA and fewer SFA: heart disease. Cholesterol and triglycerides are fats in your blood that your doctor uses as an index to show how clogged your arteries are with fatty deposits. These deposits, more appropriately called sludge, consist of a number of materials, but cholesterol is one of the major components. So, your doctor wants you to maintain both low cholesterol and low triglycerides, since the triglycerides contribute to the sludge as well.

The world's health scientists recognize that the lower your blood cholesterol and triglycerides, the less likely you are to be depositing sludge on your arterial walls. There are a number of steps you can take to reduce cholesterol; two of them are to eat a diet that's low in fat and let the fat be more PUFA than SFA with a generous complement of MFA.

There are many other things that help to reduce sludge accumulation, and we'll talk about all of them in this book.

Three we've already covered; more PUFA and MFA than SFA; don't be overweight; exercise. In subsequent chapters we'll cover fiber and other factors.

How high should your cholesterol and triglycerides be? Cholesterol, triglycerides, blood sugar and many other blood components are expressed as so many milligrams in 100 milliliters of blood. It conveniently allows the use of milligram percent and usually works with whole numbers between 50 and about 300. It is so widely practiced that we often simply use the number. Therefore, it's very likely you'll hear cholesterol expressed as, for example, 180. It really means 180 milligram percent.

Age	Cholesterol	Triglycerides
Less than 50	Less than 180 mg. %	Less than 100 mg. %
Over 50	Less than 215 mg. %	Less than 130 mg. %

Balance SFA and PUFA

In fact, we can be even more precise about the fat content of our diet. We should strive to balance SFA with PUFA. And if it is unbalanced in any direction, let it be toward PUFA.

Monounsaturated fats, like olive oil, are ideal for many reasons, so it is felt by most health professionals that they should constitute the major part of our fat intake.

Which Fats Are Best?

I can let you decide by giving you the information. The following table, from Harvard Medical School, shows the composition of commonly used fats and oils.

Oil/Fat	% SFA	% MFA	% PUFA
Coconut	92	6	2
Corn	13	25	62
Cottonseed	27	18	55
*Olive	14	77	9
Palm	53	38	9
Peanut	18	48	34
Safflower	9	13	78
Sesame	14	42	44
Soybean	15	25	60
Sunflower	11	21	68
Butter	68	28	4
Lard	41	43	16
Soft margarine	19	53	28
Shortening	25	68	7

*Considered by many to be the best all-around oil.

How Much Total Fat?

Total fat intake should not exceed 30% of calories and I propose you keep yours to 25% of calories. Now you know why nutritionists are criticized. How can I expect you to put that information to work on an everyday basis? I can't, and I don't, but give me a minute to explain.

At this point in the book I only want you to realize that there are many dietary factors that can help you normalize your blood pressure. I know you can't work with the notion of 25% to 30% of total calories as fat. After all, it doesn't identify today's lunch or tomorrow's dinner for you.

In the next part of this book you'll see how these concepts reduce to a series of *dos, don'ts,* and *occasionallys.* Then, we'll put them into some menu patterns and it will all emerge as food that you eat. You'll be able to put the concepts into meals and snacks.

Garlic

Folklore teaches that garlic cures "hot blood." "Hot blood" was not a way of describing the aggressive intentions of a Latin lover; it was terminology for what we recognize today as high blood pressure. Other plants, mostly similar to garlic, like onions and some peppers, are also purported to have this property. And on the Caribbean islands, the leaves of a bush are used for the same purpose.

I am a student of folklore. One of my previous books, *Making the Vitamin Connection* (Harper and Row, 1985), was written to show how folklore, specifically "old wives' tales," were actually the means of passing nutritional knowledge from one generation to the next. When folklore teaches something, I listen. And, with garlic, I have been rewarded.

Garlic contains one or more chemicals that resemble other chemicals, specifically a prostaglandin that each cell of your body manufactures. These prostaglandins have a significant effect on blood pressure, and knowledge of them helps us to understand why garlic was so important in preventing and curing "hot blood."

The Prostaglandins

"Prostaglandin" was the name given to a component of human semen that stimulates certain muscles to contract. We know today there are three prostaglandins. We don't store them, but every cell of your body can make them on demand if the raw materials are present. They have profound effects on human health, especially under certain conditions.

Two prostaglandins have important roles in blood pressure. The first, designated PG2, is made from either of two fatty acids, linoleic acid or arachidonic acid. Linoleic acid is a polyunsaturated fat obtained from plants and arachidonic acid is converted from linoleic acid by animals. That is why linoleic acid is designated "essential." It is required for the synthesis of arachidonic acid that is then converted to prostaglandin number two (PG2).

The other important prostaglandin, PG3, is made from a unique fatty acid appropriately named eicosapentaenoic acid, or EPA for short. EPA is in a unique class of polyunsaturated fatty acids called the omega-3 fatty acids because of their detailed structure. EPA is found in the chloroplasts of green plants, but the best source of EPA is from blue-skinned cold-water fish such as mackerel, salmon, and trout.

Although I haven't discussed how prostaglandins help prevent high blood pressure or help reduce it once established, we can draw some dietary conclusions. People with high blood pressure and people who want to maintain their normal blood pressure should be sure their diet contains both linoleic acid and EPA. That translates to lots of vegetables, vegetable oil, and fish, especially cold-water fish. In the case of EPA, supplements are appropriate for people who don't eat fish regularly.

What Do the Prostaglandins Do?

Prostaglandins, especially PG2 from linoleic acid, are important to the tone of the muscle cells that line the peripheral arterioles. This means that if the muscle cells are contracted, peripheral resistance increases and blood pressure goes up. So, you should be sure you get sufficient linoleic acid from vegetables and vegetable oils.

Drugs that inhibit prostaglandin production such as aspirin or indomethacin increase blood pressure by increasing total peripheral resistance. This tells a biochemist that the prostaglandins made from linoleic acid are involved in the dilation of the peripheral arterioles. But more, it also tells us that they will facilitate blood flow in the kidney.

They are also involved in facilitating the release of materials that help the kidneys remove sodium from the blood. Therefore, impaired production of prostaglandin from linoleic acid is not good. In fact, it will very likely contribute to if not cause high blood pressure.

The prostaglandin made from EPA is different. It doesn't have the same specific influence on peripheral resistance or on the kidney. It is required to balance the prostaglandin from linoleic acid. On the other hand, the raw material for this prostaglandin, EPA, does seem to have a specific effect.

EPA—Nature's Teflon

EPA and other omega-3 fatty acids become a part of blood cells and the cells that line the arteries and arterioles. In these positions, they act as a natural lubricant to facilitate the flow of cells through the vessels and capillaries. In this way, people who have adequate EPA usually have lower blood pressure than people who don't.

A major military research study is currently underway that reduces total fat intake and increases EPA intake in volunteers with high blood pressure. The research is showing quite well that EPA helps to reduce total peripheral resistance and contributes significantly to blood pressure reduction.

People in this study take fish oil capsules. In fact, they take from 8 to 18 capsules each containing 180 milligrams of EPA. In addition, the fish oil in the capsules contains 240 milligrams of another oil called DHA. We aren't sure how these oils reduce blood pressure, but they do. Very precise measurements indicate that these oils simply make the blood flow more easily. My analogy—nature's Teflon—is pretty good until a better explanation is found.

Folklore, Nobel Prizes, and Diet

In 1982, three distinguished scientists were awarded the Nobel Prize for their work in elucidating the workings of the prostaglandins. Indeed, this research is continuing, and someday derivatives of the prostaglandins will help reduce blood pressure in people with impaired prostaglandin production.

But now, food is still the only "natural" approach, and it dictates that we eat a diet with lots of variety. This variety should include lots of fish, vegetables, and natural condiments like garlic and onions.

How Much Fish Oil?

I recommend that we should strive for about 2 grams of fish oil daily, including about 500 milligrams of EPA. This means that if you eat cold-water blue-skinned fish about twice weekly, you'll be getting enough. On the other hand, you can obtain it from supplements (not including cod liver oil). In my opinion, about 3 capsules daily would be fine. They provide about 500 milligrams of EPA and a similar level of the similar fatty acid, DHA. This translates to 1 gram daily of these fatty acids.

You will read that some scientists are very cautious about these fish oil capsules. They are generally basing their caution on the enormous levels of 18 or more used in clinical studies. Some also point out, erroneously, that these oils contain cholesterol. In the early years, these supplements did; now they don't. In summary, at the levels I recommend, these supplements can do a great deal of good and no harm.

Chapter Eight

High Blood Pressure Origins V:
The Role of Your Kidneys

Get to Know Your Kidneys

We are born with two kidneys, each one about the size of an adult fist, located in the abdomen just under the back muscles. We can function quite well on one kidney. Since we've got two, intuition suggests they're important, because excess capacity is nature's way of insuring survival.

Within each kidney there are millions of specialized cells called nephrons. Each nephron is a marvelous filtering system. Millions of nephrons working together make a filtering system with incredible capacity. The kidneys' ability to filter sodium from the blood and regulate fluid levels is one of the three systems of blood pressure regulation in the body. Indeed, the kidneys process about 50 gallons of fluid daily.

Kidneys influence blood pressure by regulating fluid volume, including blood, and controlling the amount of sodium, potassium, calcium, and probably magnesium, in our system. In previous chapters, you learned that these minerals can profoundly influence the tenseness or relaxation of the muscles in the arterioles. So, indirectly, the kidneys affect peripheral resistance.

How Do They Do All This?

An enormous amount of blood passes through the kidneys and much fluid is removed. Then, wastes are kept out and the remaining materials, including most of the water, are returned to the blood. Waste products and the liquid that contains them are urine.

Most of the sodium and water that are removed get reabsorbed from the nephrons and returned to the blood. If there's an excess of sodium and fluid volume, the kidney cannot eliminate it. Blood pressure is elevated to overcome this situation and literally force sodium out. This process, analogous to a water-purifying system, is called reverse osmosis. But, if sodium didn't get reabsorbed, the problem wouldn't exist.

How Does Sodium Get Reabsorbed?

Sodium gets reabsorbed as sodium chloride. That's right; it gets reabsorbed into the blood as common table salt. This ability to reabsorb sodium probably evolved as a mechanism to conserve sodium and chloride, but in our modern world, it works against us because now the two elements are consumed to serious excess.

Reabsorption of sodium as sodium chloride can work against us because it causes blood pressure to be diet related. Most processed foods utilize large quantities of salt; if that's not enough, people often liberally add salt to food. Potassium supplements often consist of potassium chloride, making some situations worse. In Chapter Six you met Charlie, whose doctor thought he could reduce Charlie's blood pressure by restoring potassium–sodium balance with potassium supplements. Charlie's supplement was potassium chloride. So, while he helped the potassium level, he also helped conserve all his sodium by reabsorption to conserve the chloride.

Sodium by itself and chloride by itself in natural foods

are probably not a problem. Natural foods contain sodium in a myriad of forms including some sodium chloride. For example, sodium is found as the acetate, citrate, and gluta-mate. As a result, natural foods are naturally balanced in the forms of the sodium they contain. And they don't impose an excess of either sodium or chloride. In fact, the amount of chloride in the diet, with the body's ability to reabsorb 99% of sodium, dictates that very little dietary sodium is actually required. Normal active adults get along well on about 300 milligrams of sodium daily, and some experts claim even less is all right.

Why Reabsorb Sodium and Not Potassium?

Sodium reabsorption illustrates the body's excellent abil-ity to conserve nutrients. Salt, sodium chloride, was so scarce just 2,000 years ago that it was a medium of exchange—it was money! In fact, as recently as the Roman Empire, soldiers were paid with a salt ration. This salt ration evolved into the word "salary."

When man was roaming the African plains millions of years ago, the only sodium and chloride came from the food he ate. Since food, especially vegetable food, contains much more potassium than sodium, and not much chloride, there was no need to conserve potassium. Since sodium and chloride were both scarce, the elaborate reabsorption sys-tem in the kidneys evolved to conserve them.

In the intervening 3 or 4 million years, sodium chloride remained scarce. Only in the last 1,000 years has salt be-come readily available. And only in the last 400 years has it become cheap. In the evolutionary process, 100,000 years is a "blink of the eye," let alone 2,000. In short, man's the same, but the availability of salt has changed.

About two thirds of people don't get dramatically ele-vated blood pressure from excess sodium and reduced po-tassium. That suggests that in the distant future, our kidneys will adapt to this man-made imbalance between sodium and potassium.

One nagging last word of caution should prevail, however. In populations whose diet is natural and contains a potassium–sodium ration of 3 or more, blood pressure doesn't elevate with age. This implies that as part of the aging process, we lose the ability to handle excess sodium chloride in our diet because our blood pressure increases with age. Therefore, until we know better, it is sensible for everyone to maintain a potassium to sodium ratio of 3 or more. But it seems equally and perhaps more important to reduce the intake of sodium chloride.

Hormonal Influence

Kidneys are under the influence of a number of hormonal systems. All of these hormones, when not functioning properly or in synchrony, seem to cause sodium reabsorption. They can be influenced by diet or drugs, so let me walk you through them.

Insulin was discussed in Chapter Five. Excess insulin causes sodium reabsorption by the kidney, indirectly elevating blood pressure. This makes people who produce excess insulin candidates for high blood pressure. Consequently, many overweight people, people who habitually consume excess sugar, and some diabetics who do not control insulin correctly, develop high blood pressure.

Another more elaborate hormone system that influences blood pressure is the angiotensin-renin-aldosterone system. This system includes the adrenal glands, which produce aldosterone, the primary hormone that induces the kidneys to retain sodium and chloride and excrete potassium. Aldosterone is produced by the two adrenal glands, which are situated on top of each kidney.

Aldosterone causes the kidney and the sweat glands (which act, to some extent, like kidneys) to retain sodium. Although aldosterone is produced by the adrenal glands, it is, in part, regulated by events in the kidney. This regulation involves the hormone angiotensin and the enzyme renin.

Kidneys release renin, an enzyme that causes the release of another hormone, angiotensin. Angiotensin causes constriction of the arterioles and this signals the adrenals to release more aldosterone. It follows from what we've discussed that constriction of the arterioles and the release of aldosterone elevates blood pressure by two mechanisms. Arteriole constriction causes increased peripheral resistance and aldosterone causes salt retention. So we'd better examine renin production.

Renin is produced by stimulation of the sympathetic nervous system. This is the nervous system that takes charge during fright. If someone attacks you, either mentally or physically, your kidneys release renin and the entire angiotensin-aldosterone process is started. This takes our blood pressure discussion into the realm of stress, which we'll discuss in the next chapter.

Some physicians who specialize in hypertension talk of "high renin producers." High-renin producers are people, often with Type A personalities (Chapter Nine), who normally produce excess renin. Excess renin leads to elevated blood pressure. In some cases the only recourse is to control renin levels with drugs that block its production.

A small amount of evidence suggests that inadequate magnesium can cause excessive renin production. There is no excuse for inadequate magnesium, since we can either get it from food or from food supplements.

Before leaving the renin-angiotensin-aldosterone system, I should point out that some serious conditions can cause excessive aldosterone. These are serious illnesses that must be dealt with by modern medical intervention. In these cases the blood pressure is secondary to the illness and cannot be dealt with by diet.

There are other factors not as well understood that influence the rate of sodium excretion by the kidneys. These materials, appropriately called natriuretic factors (meaning sodium excretion factors), are produced in other parts of the body and influence the way the kidneys handle sodium. Natriuretic factors are produced in response to increased blood sodium levels; therefore, diets high or low in sodium will influence their levels proportionately.

Putting All This Together: You're In Control

Your kidneys are incredible! They are responsible for cleansing the blood of waste materials, but even more important, they can, to varying degrees, produce high blood pressure. But, barring a disease that causes excess renin production, this capacity is under dietary control! Therefore, they can equally be envisioned as organs of prevention.

Kidney-induced high blood pressure is related to excessive sodium chloride. It's possibly made even worse by excessive chloride, which can even come from potassium chloride. Natural sodium or potassium salts from food do not contribute excessive chloride. The sodium chloride problem can be regulated by diet. In this sense, we are what we eat. And excessive salt sets the stage for high blood pressure. So, reducing total salt intake is important.

A secondary issue involves insulin, as discussed in Chapter Five. But insulin excess is the result of overweight or poor dietary habits. Overweight is under our control even though weight loss is often not easy, and excessive sugar consumption is a matter of dietary control.

A later chapter is devoted to reducing salt, but you can start right now. It's easy: Reduce consumption of processed foods and start reading ingredient lists. Try to eliminate everything that has salt on the ingredient list.

Processed foods contain salt either as a preservative or to increase taste intensity, or perhaps a technologist has added it because it's the thing to do. Return to natural foods, fruits, grains, vegetables, meat, fish, poultry—anything that grew from the ground, on the ground, on trees, walked, swam, or flew. Do not prepare or eat anything with elaborate sauces or coatings. Boil, broil, barbecue, bake, or poach without adding salt. It works!

At first you might say the food's bland, but in a short time, you'll begin to enjoy your increased taste sensitivity. You'll start savoring flavors that you didn't know were present. A new world of taste will open to you.

Dealing with stress is also important, because it can lead to excess renin production. Although this is not strictly a dietary issue, it is one variable that we can control and must be dealt with as a lifestyle issue.

Chapter Nine

High Blood Pressure Origins VI:
Stress

Colonel Oliver's Story

Visualize an examining room in the Pentagon medical clinic. Air Force Colonel Oliver, stripped to the waist, is nearing the end of his annual physical. The examining physician is talking with him and the phone buzzes. The doctor takes the call, speaks to a voice at the other end, and looks at Colonel Oliver. "It's for you, your adjutant, and he says it's urgent." He hands over the phone.

As Oliver spoke into the telephone, the doctor saw anxiety, dismay, and fear cover his face. He realized that the man in front of him was experiencing extreme mental stress. He took a bold step, grabbed a syringe, took Oliver's arm, and extracted a blood sample. The colonel was on the phone for 20 minutes; the doctor got two samples. With the blood he had taken during the physical, he had three samples: one before, one at the beginning of the event, and one after Oliver was about 15 minutes into the stress. The doctor took blood pressure and pulse simultaneously with an electronic sphygmomanometer.

In the last years of the twentieth century it's easy to understand Colonel Oliver's stress. His adjutant explained to him that he had been charged, by a responsible Washington reporter, with misappropriating funds to a major Air

Force contractor. The accusations were so serious that, if founded, they could destroy Oliver's fine career. He was an Academy graduate, a decorated Vietnam pilot, and destined to wear at least one general's star before retirement—if the reporter didn't terminate his career that afternoon.

Oliver's stress was of the worst kind. He was trapped in circumstances and location where he couldn't do anything about the situation until he returned to his office and marshalled his resources.

You might ask, "If he's not guilty, why would he experience stress?"

In Washington, issues are usually vague and don't die. Colonel Oliver's innocence could be proven in court, but his "real" trial would take place in the court of public opinion, and that could rule the day. After all, in these times, a general officer must be a politician, diplomat, contractor, and sometimes a fighting man.

Colonel Oliver's Blood Results

Oliver is a fine physical specimen; 6'0", 185 pounds. He maintains excellent condition by running and working out daily. Many men could take lessons from him.

Before the call, his resting pulse rate was 56 while sitting. His doctor's first measurement, about 5 minutes into the call, showed a pulse of about 84; 15 minutes later, it was about 96. His blood pressure at rest was 110/70; 5 minutes into the call, it was 130/85; 15 minutes into the call, it was 140/95.

Blood chemistry at 5 minutes showed twice normal levels of adrenaline in his blood. His blood sugar had gone from a normal of 80 milligrams to about 100, and there was a rise in the free fatty acids. Fifteen minutes into the call, the adrenaline was more elevated, blood sugar was at 100, free fatty acids were 25% above normal, and even his blood cholesterol was 10% higher than before the call.

What Can We Learn from Colonel Oliver?

If Colonel Oliver were going to fly into combat, or run five miles, or engage in some other physical activity, he'd be ready! In short, he was ready to fight or to retreat; and the colonel doesn't have "retreat" in his vocabulary. All he could do was have his adjutant pull the appropriate files and notify the correct people of the situation. Hopefully, Oliver could sit with the reporter and by showing appropriate information convince him diplomatically of his erroneous conclusions.

His blood chemistry tells us quite clearly that Colonel Oliver's body was ready to deal with stress physically. But that would not happen unless he wanted a jail sentence. In contrast, all he could do was try to control the situation by balancing the facts with rhetoric and persuasion. And he could only hope the affair would not leave a bad taste in people's minds.

What About His Body?

Science tells us that when people are faced with this type of stress regularly, they are more likely to have high blood pressure. There seems to be a type of adaptation that takes place—a sort of negative adaptation.

You know from the previous chapter that the colonel's kidneys released renin and the renin-angiotensin-aldosterone system went to work. This caused his body to retain sodium and constrict his peripheral arterioles. In short, it prepared the colonel to fight.

By increasing peripheral resistance, his brain (the main organ) gets more blood. Higher pulse means more blood flow. Elevated blood sugar provides short-term energy; elevated free fatty acids provide energy for him to go a couple of hours. Increased adrenaline meant that his energy level would remain elevated for hours. He didn't sleep that night!

It would have been best for Colonel Oliver if, after in-structing his adjutant, he could have run about five miles. The run would burn off the extra energy, let the adrenaline stabilize, relax his peripheral arterioles and return every-thing, including blood pressure, to normal. But he couldn't do that. If this kind of event occurred regularly, Oliver would either find a way to deal with it or it would effect him physically with high blood pressure.

Some scientists would argue that the increase in blood pressure is the outcome of subtle behavioral changes made by the person under stress. Overeating, excessive alcohol, not finding time for exercise (like Frank in Chapter One), are just a few possible stress-related behavioral changes. Other equally learned scientists argue that elevated blood pressure results from this so-called negative adaptation that takes place, and slowly maintains the body in a "ready" to fight state.

Other Examples of Stress

While Colonel Oliver's study was anecdotal, that is, the report of one event, there have been studies that verify the reality of his experience. For example, high blood pressure is endemic in air traffic controllers. But I like to use two examples that most people can readily visualize. One comes from racing car drivers and another from doctors.

Racing Drivers: Conditioned to Stress

Three minutes before the race, drivers sit in their cars while mechanics make last-minute preparations. Before the engines are started, changes in blood composition start. Adrenaline is released, blood sugar is elevated, and free fatty acids are released. This is before engines are even started. Things are quiet. All the changes are the result of mental anticipation of the short-term future.

One minute before the race, as the order to "start engines" goes out, pulse rates quicken, blood pressure increases significantly, and adrenaline is even higher. It's no longer mental; its real!

During the race, all these factors stabilize at a level that is elevated, but normal for the circumstances. "Circumstances" in this case means driving around a 2.5-mile track at speeds ranging from 150 to 200 miles per hours and more. Reactions must be instantaneous and energy levels high. Mistakes often mean serious injury or death.

Do the changes sound familiar? They are no different than what Colonel Oliver went through. But the drivers are conditioned to it; they are prepared. Oliver wasn't.

These world-class drivers have raced so often that three minutes before the start their internal clock tells them that "controlled pandemonium" will occur in three minutes. Their bodies respond by producing the substances that get blood flowing to the brain, provide the short- and long-term energy needed to fight or run or, in this case, compete.

In contrast, Colonel Oliver's body sensed the same impending fight and prepared for it, but had nowhere to go. Colonel Oliver could only box at shadows, not at real people.

The Doctors: "It's All Relative"

Several doctors were asked to prepare and deliver a talk on patient care to separate groups of physicians and nurses. They went to give the same talk, without change. The difference was predictable. While delivering the talk to his peers, the group of physicians, each doctor's pulse rate quickened, his blood pressure increased, and changes in blood chemistry occurred. The reaction was most obvious during the question session.

In contrast, the nurse audience did not elicit such a response. During the doctors' speeches, pulse and blood pressure were normal for anyone standing and speaking, such as a teacher. The question session was no different than the rest of the session.

This tells us that stressful situations are relative to the circumstances. Peer group doctors can have a significant influence on a doctor's career; in contrast, nurses generally do not. It is no surprise then that the audience of physicians caused more significant reactions.

An Analysis of External Stress

Stress undoubtedly influences our body, and it's proportional to the situation and potential outcome. Indeed, the changes that occur in our blood have probably been the same for tens of thousands of years. In short, it's the old "fight or flight" situation—a term first coined by Dr. Hans Selye, an expert on stress.

What we do about it is important, though. If race car drivers can condition for stress, why can't we all? We can!

In Colonel Oliver's case, he was already conditioned. The best thing for him, after getting the adjutant started on his defense, would have been to jog five miles, then arrange a meeting with the reporter, and steadfastly maintain his health program no matter how bad the ordeal became. I should add, quite happily, that he did jog that day, and he successfully presented evidence in his defense to the reporter at breakfast the next morning. I still predict he will be a general before he retires.

Air traffic controllers have endemic high blood pressure, most likely because they are sedentary, smoke, and take out their frustrations with poor eating and drinking habits. In short, stress is only the initiator. In the final analysis, it's diet and lifestyle that affect their blood pressure.

Race car drivers deal with stress effectively. They are excellent examples of how mental stress can be used to advantage by the body, but more important, how the body prepares for physical stress. If the drivers would practice the diet and lifestyle programs in this book, they'd do great.

In contrast to all this, the doctors' study teaches us that stress is relative. In a later chapter, we'll talk about the power of positive thinking. If the doctors had practiced positive thinking, they would have been as relaxed in front of their peers as in front of the nurses.

Internally Generated Stress

Colonel Oliver, race car drivers, and the doctors I described all faced extreme forms of external stress. With logic or conditioning, they could learn to deal with it. But, there's another much more insidious and deadly kind of stress: It's "internally generated stress," which we create ourselves.

Internally generated stress starts at an early age. Some of it is hereditary, some is learned from our parents, but at some point this stress can consume one's personality. It can create a tense, unrelaxing person with "tense" or "uptight" characteristics.

Dealing with Stress

Whether stress is internal or external, there are things we can do to gain control. We can condition for stress in several ways, and I have devoted a chapter to it. But for now, remember three critical things.

1. Don't try to relieve the frustration caused by stress by creating more stress. Don't drink, snack, smoke, or use chemicals. Tranquilizers will never prevent high blood pressure!
2. Maintain fitness. A conditioned, nonoverweight body copes well with stress.

3. Mental conditioning for external stress is equally important. Prepare for the "worst" eventually and decide how you would handle it. Once you're ready, what actually occurs will be easy.

Type A and Type B Behavior

I am proud to have Dr. Martin Friedman's autograph in my visitor's book. He revolutionized thinking on behavior when he identified two personality types: type A and type B. Based on his books and about 20 years of dealing with people, I determine the two types this way. Have a conversation with someone on a mutually appealing subject and observe what happens as you talk. Type A people will finish your sentence for you if you seem to slow down or search your mind to make a point. Type B people will relax, let you make your point, nod in agreement, and slowly discuss their opposing view.

Dr. Friedman and others have extensively studied these differences in people and have concluded that behavior type influences our health dramatically. They teach that Type A personality is much more prone to heart attacks and high blood pressure. Type A's lead a life that is always tense and in constant frustration of wanting to do more, be better, and get ahead.

Type A personalities are characterized by many traits. I will summarize a few of them for you as succinctly as possible.

- Vocal explosiveness characterized by emphasizing key words and finishing sentences quickly.
- Impatience with the pace of things. They walk, talk, and eat rapidly, unconsciously urging things forward by saying things to force conclusions or showing irritation.

- Polyphasic behavior, i.e., doing several things at one time. For example, a Type A person can be caught reading something out of the corner of her eye while someone is speaking.
- Observation is reduced to the point of not noticing things. For example, a Type A's visit to someone's home or office produces no recall of surroundings, only the conversation.
- Chronic time urgency to the point of working very long hours and still constantly falling behind. Type A people often try to do more and more in less and less time.
- Obsessive tendency to reduce everything to the "numbers."
- Compulsive competitiveness with others, especially fellow Type A personalities. Instead of attempting to work with other Type A's, they compete with each other. They seem to see everyone as a challenge.

Obviously, personality traits are complex and not easily defined, but from the above, you can get a feeling for Type A behavior. It's compulsive and characterized by a sense of urgency. Type B personalities are at the other extreme. The laid-back Type B doesn't tend to get high blood pressure, because he's relaxed, content with himself, and works hard but takes plenty of time to "smell the roses."

Type B personalities are easy to characterize by contrast. The Type B personality knows his own virtues and makes do with what he's got. His personality is best characterized by the cartoon character Popeye, who said, "I am what I am and that's all that I am, I'm Popeye the sailor man." Let me summarize Type B behavior for you.

- Free of Type A traits, especially the overpowering sense of urgency.

- Not impatient.
- No anxiety, no free-floating hostility, an ability to relax without guilt, work without agitation.
- Able to play and work without competing with everyone.

The Type B personality is not to be confused with under-achievement. Type B's can be just as accomplished in life; there's simply a difference in how they do things. They are comfortable with themselves and can accomplish without competition. They lack the sense of time urgency that characterizes the compulsive Type A.

It's important to recognize that very few personalities are completely Type A or Type B. Further, we all have aspects of each within us, but from these a general picture emerges that, for simplicity, we classify as either A or B.

How Does Type A Affect High Blood Pressure?

Type A people are always tense. In Chapter Two, Bill, the man with nosebleeds, is an absolute Type A. When I'm with him, I visualize a tightly coiled spring across from me. He's no fun to be with, and you can't relax in his presence because his tenseness is contagious. The only people who like him are as tense or more tense than he.

It's not surprising that Bill has high blood pressure. After all, his total peripheral resistance to blood flow is always elevated. I suspect that a specialist would find that Bill is a high renin producer, and we know from the previous chapter that that's a cause of high blood pressure. His tenseness elevates his blood pressure because about 3 million years of evolution have made us respond that way. I've never seen any evidence that allows me to believe that we should try to alter this normal response chemically with tranquilizers, alcohol, or other substances, unless it is clear that there's no other way.

Lunch with Bill

Bill is Type A; lunch with him is like dining with a coiled spring. He's definitely not overweight; in fact, he appears a little underweight. And he eats a lot of high-fat food. Let me correct myself, he "inhales" a lot of high-fat food; he's usually finished and having his coffee when I'm in the middle of my meal. Let me describe a lunch with Bill.

What was going to be a private lunch ended at a large, loud restaurant where you must sit at tables that also have four other people around them. Having a quick, private conversation is simply not possible. Bill's at home there. He ordered two large frankfurters with sauerkraut and German potatoes. He inhaled them while I was attempting to discuss some issues over the din that prevailed in the place. Bill had German chocolate cake and two cups of coffee by the time I finished my halibut and salad. I didn't have coffee; in fact, I drink tea. But I prefer to have it quietly later in the afternoon. On the way back to Bill's office, he stopped for a café latté at a sidewalk shop and drank it on the way.

So here we are walking down the street after he has inhaled a high-fat, high-salt lunch with a high-calorie, high-sodium dessert, followed by two cups of coffee. And then he stops for more coffee to drink while walking! No wonder he has high blood pressure.

I submit that it's impossible to separate out the origins of his high blood pressure. His diet probably has at least twice as much sodium as potassium. His lunches, and I've had many with him, consist of at least 50% of calories from fat. Then there are the three cups of coffee, that's 300 to 400 milligrams of caffeine within 90 minutes. His body will require at least three hours to cope with that much caffeine.

I have also met Bill for breakfast. He similarly inhales that meal and it usually consists of fried eggs, bacon or sausage, hash browns, and coffee. Always eaten in a rush, he usually drinks coffee on the walk back to work.

Bill is a complete Type A; his personality not only influences how he deals with others, but it also pervades his entire life. A meeting with him is always rushed. Even if he has time, he looks at his watch often and gives other signals of time pressure, such as finishing sentences for others, or even telling them to get to the bottom line. Once, sailing with him on a somewhat calm day, it became obvious he was impatient with the light breeze even though we had nothing important to do and the entire day to do it in. In fact, I once had lunch with him in a private club where they don't serve franks and sauerkraut. He had fish, but with a rich sauce, more coffee, and dessert. And would you believe it, he stopped for coffee to drink as we walked back!

Barry's Story

I worked with a man named Barry who once held the same position as Bill and was also Type A. I emphasize *was*; although I know he still has Type A traits, he has channeled them effectively.

Barry was so typical Type A it dominated his life. It determined the location of his home, left his first marriage in shambles, and led him to be overweight; in short, he lost track of himself on the way to the top. No one could explain anything to him. I watched two to three of my colleagues get fired by him each year. My survival strategy was to stay clear and duck below the level of fire.

But Barry was also the man who personally introduced me to Dr. Friedman. Barry made a conscious effort to deal with his behavior as a result of Dr. Friedman and his book *Type A Behavior and Your Heart*. Let me tell you what he's done:

Barry exercises daily. He jogs, or uses a stationary bike,

or swims at his private club. And he works his upper body on resistance bars so his conditioning is complete. He has a well-rounded program.

Breakfast is usually fruit and yogurt, and one cup of coffee. In ten years, I have never seen him eat eggs, bacon, or sausage.

Lunch is most often a salad, fish, or a pasta dish with a non-meat sauce. If he has dessert, it is fresh fruit; then one cup of coffee, but often it's tea.

Dinner is light. No red meat, usually fish or poultry, wine in moderation, a light dessert, and tea, if any stimulant at all.

When I first met Barry, he finished every sentence I started; he seldom let anyone else speak. After working with experts (including me) he learned to listen, to think before he spoke, and to read a lot more than he ever had before.

He shared the result of his recent annual physical with me. He's in excellent health—not as good as me—but excellent nonetheless. (Even Type B's can be competitive sometimes!)

Barry still uses his Type A traits to get ahead. He's now worth over seven million dollars and growing. But he has successfully controlled his Type A behavior, and directed it toward his business life. He follows an excellent diet and lifestyle pattern and smells the roses. He'll live a long, healthy life.

A Tale of Two Type A's

Both Bill and Barry have similar impatient, tense, and competitive personalities. Perhaps that's what it takes to get where they are. Both of them let their drive consume their lives totally. But Barry recognized what he was doing to himself and he took charge. He's a pleasure to be with now when he's "off duty," because he's relaxed and easy to converse with. In contrast, I don't know anyone who enjoys being with Bill. Indeed, his Type A traits continue to dominate every aspect of his life. I hope some day someone can get through to him before the rest of his health deteriorates. If he'll follow Barry's cue, his troubles are over. His health will be restored and his good qualities can emerge. Lunch with him will no longer be an ordeal.

Type A or B: Does It Matter?

Although debate about this will continue, I think it does matter whether you are Type A or Type B. But, I think your personality behavior matters for reasons that are not causative, but contributory. Both types can get high blood pressure. You met Gene in Chapter Two; he's as much a Type B as anyone can be—remember, it was Gene who was passive about the loss of his sex life. Frank (from Chapter One) is more B than A. Clearly Barry is Type A, and Bill makes many Type A's look like Type B's by comparison.

Barry's Type A personality led him to be as aggressive about his health as he is about his work. I deeply believe the change in diet and lifestyle has given him a new lease on a more abundant life. Sure, he's still the aggressive businessman, but he listens as hard as he bargains. He's doing better in business for it. He actively makes time for his family and his second wife. They are well suited for each other because she likes the Type A life, in contrast to his first wife who didn't. And, as I write this, he and his family are on a one-week river rafting trip in the Grand Canyon. Barry has successfully channeled his Type A traits to improve the quality of his life . . . and the lives of everyone he loves.

Gene's Type B behavior works against him. He accepts things too easily, and lives a life of quiet desperation. Until I booted him into action, he was willing to give up the pleasure of sex. How passive can you get? But, he has a lot going for him. Once his blood pressure is under non-drug control, he has the advantage of not having Type A traits, so he doesn't have to overcome the coiled spring syndrome that typifies Bill. But Gene needs someone to make sure he eats correctly and a vigilant doctor to watch that he doesn't slip back into the old, comfortable rut.

Frank is somewhere in between A and B. Dr. Friedman would place him pretty close to the middle. He's an aggressive businessman, but can't control himself enough to follow a diet. He's like many people who seem to have been programmed to have food and lifestyle dictated by someone else. Usually we eat what we were raised to like, or we comfortably eat whatever our spouses, friends, or kids are eating. It's hard to buck a trend. Consequently, Frank's doctor probably needs to deal directly with Frank's wife so she can help Frank make the right food and lifestyle decisions. We'll see in a subsequent chapter that he can learn to take control with a few simple techniques.

From the above, you must realize that I believe it doesn't matter what personality type you are—anyone can get high blood pressure. I think that if personality is a factor, Type A's are most likely to get high blood pressure. But what really counts is what they do about it. I can see a clear, positive approach either way.

Know Thyself

First try and decide whether you're Type A or Type B. It's fun to ask yourself some questions and get an idea of how you behave.

1. Do you consider yourself an aggressive driver? A workaholic? Are you proud of it?
2. Do you feel anxious when you are not working? Like you should be doing something task oriented?
3. Are you thinking of the next project while one is still underway?

4. Do you compete with everyone around you? Are you always trying to get ahead?
5. Do people take notice of how much work you do? Are you known for long hours of hard work?
6. Do you listen to people, let them express themselves? Do you finish sentences for them?

I am sure that you can design other questions yourself. Better still, ask some people around you. Ask a colleague who has no commitment to your career or your job; you may be surprised at what you learn.

We'll return to behavioral modification in a later chapter. Now use some common sense and make a list of things you should change, regardless of your type. Some suggestions:

- Set aside more time for exercise and leisure activities.
- Save more time for directed activities with loved ones.
- Plan a diet from what this book will teach. Get control of your physical health.
- Plan a realistic exercise program from this and other books, and put it into action.
- Examine the chapter on weight and take the "bag" test to see how much work you've got to do.

I'm sure you can think of many more changes. Your personality type doesn't matter. If you were using your Type A behavior as an excuse, such as "I was born tense," you were simply rationalizing your life away. Take charge as either type and do whatever is necessary to get your health in order.

Additional Reading

Type A Behavior and Your Heart
Friedman, M., M.D., and Rosenman R. H., M.D.
Fawcett, 1974, 4th Printing, 1985

Section Two

Foods and Recipes

Prologue

Let Food Be Thy Medicine

You've come a long way and have a working knowledge of your body and why your blood pressure has become elevated. Don't think of high blood pressure as an illness; rather, think of it as a food and weight boundary you must live within. We all live within boundaries. Thankfully, most boundaries are man-made, physical, or economic, because the most restrictive boundaries are mental, created in our minds as children by well-intentioned parents, ethnic origins, teachers, people we admire, and friends. In contrast, the food boundaries handed to us by high blood pressure are easy to live with because so many alternatives are available. Indeed, the abundance of our wealthy land makes the dietary plan a sort of game rather than a restrictive lifestyle.

Begin thinking of food as Hippocrates did when he said, "Let food be thy medicine." By taking this approach, you will be able to live comfortably within your new boundaries. There's a very, very high probability that you can stop using medication altogether. If you can't stop altogether, you can reduce its use to an absolute minimum.

You will achieve complete control over your health. By controlling the nutrition foundation, you will gain a new outlook on life, realizing that however you visualize yourself, you can become. Gaining control over one factor will help you realize that you can gain control over many other factors in life. You will agree with me when I say, "As you think, you do" and "As you visualize yourself, you become."

In this section, the dietary concepts we explored will be translated into everyday food. We'll get to the bottom line—what will you have for tomorrow's breakfast, lunch, and dinner? My objective is that when you finish this part you will be able to answer that question without hesitation. But more, you will be able to enjoy the pleasures of eating and control your health.

Chapter Ten

How to Achieve Blood Pressure Control Without Drugs

Your new eating habits must accomplish several objects in order to maintain reduced blood pressure for life. You must strive to reduce sodium intake to 500 milligrams daily. Therefore, you must strive to reduce total salt intake to less than 1,300 milligrams. Your K Factor should be at least 3, preferably 4 or 5. Your food should not cause large secretions of insulin. Fat must be balanced between saturated and unsaturated, but also must provide a balance between the omega-6 PUFA from vegetables and omega-3 PUFA from fish. Your eating habits must be easy to maintain and not require planning each meal or each day like a military operation or Greek tragedy. In a word, it should come naturally.

Omega-3 and Omega-6 Fatty Acids

Omega-3 PUFA and omega-6 PUFA is scientific short-hand for a group of special polyunsaturated fatty acids (PUFA) that originate in plants. The omega-6's are readily available from most oil-bearing plants such as corn, soy, and others, while the omega-3's are found in the chloroplasts of green plants and some oil-bearing nuts including walnuts. But the best source of the major omega-3 fatty acid, eicosapenteanoic acid, EPA for short, is cold water fish.

This is because the fish eat green algae and concentrate the oil in their flesh. So EPA is obtained by eating fish, or by taking omega-3 oil supplements. Do not confuse omega-3 supplements with cod liver oil supplements. They aren't always the same.

Your diet will contain more than enough omega-6's, but is not likely to contain the omega-3's unless you eat fish regularly. That's why, throughout this book, I urge you to make fish a regular part of your diet.

Protein and Protein Quality

Adults require 45 to 65 grams of protein daily; that's about 2 or 3 ounces. Only protein supplements are "pure protein," so it's impractical to think of so many grams or ounces of pure protein. Indeed, we eat food to get protein and should only rarely use protein supplements as the sole source of protein. Common protein food sources contain up to 18% protein by weight and include fish, fowl, dairy products, beans, and other vegetables. Our objective in this plan is to obtain protein with minimal salt, minimal fat, and as much complex carbohydrate as possible. This latter objective translates to an abundant use of vegetable foods.

Amino acids are the building blocks of protein; they are the chemical units that, when bonded together, form the protein. Visualize a protein as a long string of 22 different beads that can be linked together in any number of 3 or more with no upper limit. In addition to the 22 amino acid "beads," each strand has a unique three-dimensional structure. Therefore, there is no limit to the number of proteins that can be made in nature.

Our bodies can manufacture 13 of the 22 commonly available amino acids. The 9 that we can't make are called essential because without them we cannot live. These essential amino acids must be provided by the protein we get from the food we eat. Not surprisingly, the quality of food protein is determined by the amounts of 9 essential amino acids it contains. Therefore, by designating a protein of high or low quality, we are really commenting on its amino acid composition, how many of the essential ones it provides. In general, in a diet as varied as ours, protein quality is not a problem.

Protein of animal origin, such as meat, fish, poultry, eggs, and milk, is of excellent quality. Since this plan allows all of these sources, protein quality is not an issue. If you choose to use protein supplements, their quality should be declared on the label. In addition, since you can and should eat a wide variety of protein-rich foods, any shortfall in the protein quality of one will usually be compensated for by the quality of another. Even if you should choose to become a strict vegetarian with the remote possibility of lower-quality protein, I'll show you how to mix and match vegetable sources to insure good protein quality. Therefore, this eating strategy will provide enough protein of sufficient quality to give you abundant health.

I want you to focus your attention on the sodium and potassium content of food, its K factor, and its fat content. These are the critical issues that will determine your success in controlling high blood pressure without drugs.

How Much Protein?

Adults require from 45 to 65 grams of protein depending on their size and the quality of the protein. Actually, most Americans usually get up to 100 or even 125 grams of protein daily because they eat so much meat. The excess result from our abundance of protein-rich foods. In our society, we seldom find people who do not get sufficient protein of good quality. Since there are 28 grams to an ounce, 65 grams of protein comes to just over 2 ounces of pure protein. And, since protein-rich foods such as meats and fish are about 18% protein by weight, that comes to less than 13 ounces of these protein-rich foods daily required to get enough protein for good health. Since Americans get protein of such excellent quality, 13 ounces is more than enough for most people.

The Caloric Cost of Protein

Every food provides calories. All food, including protein-rich foods, provides 4 calories from each gram of protein, 4 from each gram of carbohydrate, and 9 calories from each gram of fat. Therefore, the lower the fat content, the lower the number of calories that must be consumed to obtain protein from animal sources. This applies when comparing fish or fowl to beef, and more appropriately, processed meat as compared to fresh meat. Most vegetable sources of protein, such as beans, mushrooms, peas, and grains, contain very little fat but are rich in carbohydrates and dietary fiber. Since carbohydrate-rich foods are bulky from the digestible carbohydrate and the nondigestible fiber, you need to eat more food to obtain sufficient protein from vegetable sources. But due to the lower caloric cost of carbohydrate, eating more doesn't increase your caloric intake.

Table One
The Calorie and Sodium Cost of Protein

Our program must also compare protein sources with respect to sodium content, salt content, and the K Factor. This is easy, but it's still the old good news/bad news story.

Good news: The K Factor of meat, including fish and fowl, is usually greater than 3; more likely 5 or 6. So these foods are in.

Bad news: Processed meat of any type, sausage, cold cuts, etc., includes an incredible excess of sodium and the K Factor is unacceptable. So these foods are out.

This table compares the calories required to obtain 20

grams or about ¾ ounce of protein, about one third the daily requirement, from commonly accepted foods. The tabulation similarly illustrates the sodium content and the K Factor. *Unacceptable foods are italicized.* Averages have been compiled from standard food tables. Individual foods will vary quantitatively, but not qualitatively. Although you may find that a specific food may not be the same as the values shown here, unless it is quite unique, it should be sufficiently similar that the caloric values and K Factor will be close enough.

Food	Calories	% Calories As Fat	Sodium (mg.)	K Factor
Beef				
Sirloin, chuck, hamburger	160	31	36	6.0
Meatloaf (traditional recipe)	195	43	765	0.6
Frankfurter, bologna	456	81	1,707	0.2
Pork				
Lean ham, pork chop	175	50	48	6.5
Sausage	512	80	3,214	0.2
Game				
Rabbit	114	25	26	9.0
Venison	98	14	48	5.0
Chicken				
Chicken with skin	137	38	44	5.0
Chicken without skin	105	18	43	5.0
Chicken (frozen Stouffer's)	202	56	572	0.5
Turkey				
White meat with skin	137	38	44	5.0
White meat without skin	104	18	44	5.0
Sliced with gravy	204	25	1,925	0.2
Processed turkey ham	135	36	1,052	0.3
Processed as turkey loaf	89	14	1,270	0.2
Fish				
Fin fish (cod, blue, sea bass, tuna, flounder, salmon)	120	18	61	5.0

Food	Calories	% Calories As Fat	Sodium (mg)	K Factor
Canned tuna (oil or water packed)	86	7	386	0.7
Canned tuna (water, no salt)	86	7	47	7.0
Frozen fish sticks	212	46	216	2.2
Frozen fish sticks in batter	384	44	1,311	0.2
Lobster, crab (meat only)	107	19	83	5.0
Clams, oyster (meat only)	144	10	368	1.5
Dairy Foods				
Eggs	258	63	282	1.0
2% Milk	206	35	208	3.0
Yogurt (from skim milk)	195	3	267	3.0
Cheese (brick, cheddar, Jack, American, and Swiss)	300	71	675	0.15
Vegetables				
Beans, raw, or cooked (kidney, garbanzo)	314	6	7	150.0
Beans, canned	314	6	1,200	0.9
Pasta cooked	590	4	3	115.0
Pasta cooked with canned sauce	510	40	1,925	0.5

Guide to Table One

Most people obtain their protein from meat, fish, poultry, dairy products, including eggs, and some vegetables. You can compare the fat content of foods by examining the calories required for 20 grams of protein; that's about one third the daily requirement of 65 grams. Another important value for comparison is the percentage of calories from fat, because it's important to seek foods that have less than 30% of calories from fat. Critically important to readers of this book is to seek foods with a high K Factor. Table One shows that processing destroys it. An added bonus of this program is that processed meats with poor K Factors are often those with excessive fat. So by cutting them out, you also eliminate much fat.

Red Meat

Red meat in moderation is okay. If a low-fat cut is chosen, such as lean hamburger, shank or top round, and it is broiled, calories from fat are not excessive and the meat's K Factor is very good provided you don't add salt. Game such as rabbit and venison is outstanding.

In contrast to fresh meat, processed meats are atrocious in every respect. Their calories from fat are excessive to the point of being nutritionally obscene, and the use of salt makes bad go beyond worse. Processed meats have nothing going for them and everything against them. They are not allowed in our house or on our boat, and are never eaten by any of us in restaurants. We don't even feed them to the cat!

Poultry and Fish

In general, meat from animals that fly and swim is better than most red meat because it is lower in fat and has excellent K Factors. Crustaceans and shellfish can be a problem and require planning.

Poultry is improved by removing the skin; calories are reduced, fat is reduced, and the K Factor remains intact. But processing beyond that rears the ugly head of increased sodium and the obliteration of nature's K Factor of 3 or more. A sad testimony to food processing is turkey loaf. Turkey loaf is low in fat, but is so high in sodium that it makes sea water seem good to drink. It's the same with seafood. Simple freezing makes it convenient, but adding batter, etc., destroys the K Factor.

Dairy Products

Dairy products, including eggs, bring to the fore sodium without salt. While they contain more sodium than I prefer, it is generally in a form other than salt and that makes these foods okay if not used to excess. And their major advantage is high-quality protein without fat.

Eggs are okay. In menu planning, they should be eaten with other "balancing" foods, that is, foods rich in potassium: for example, a vegetable omelet using zucchini, mushrooms, and tomatoes. Milk is an excellent source of protein, but you might feel waterlogged from so much milk, even though you'd be healthy for the experience. Cheese, the traditional form of preserving the protein value of milk, is a disaster for anyone with high blood pressure. It will simply have to be avoided, or low-sodium cheeses sought out.

Vegetable Sources of Protein

Beans and rice together serve a large part of the world as an excellent source of protein. In fact, when made from scratch, both have very low fat, low sodium, and an excellent K Factor. But canned beans obliterate these beautiful features by adding so much salt as to be almost diabolical. Pasta, if made with a low-sodium, low-fat sauce, is excellent. In the recipe section, you will find a low-sodium sauce to preserve this fine option. On this eating plan you will be able to eat an endless variety of fresh vegetables. You will not be able to eat most canned vegetables.

Fat

About 25% to 30% of our calories should come from fat, even for active adults. Most people get about 42% of calories from fat. That excess increases the risk of cancer and heart disease, adds to elevated blood pressure, and reduces the ability for physical activity. Fat has nothing going for it and everything against it in our society. Excessive fat consumption remains a continuing problem for most people. Do something about it now. Table One helps you to identify protein sources that contain less fat. It's clear that to maintain a good K Factor, you've got to seek natural protein food such as meat, fish, and poultry. Poultry and fish contain less fat, so the obvious choice is to shift your diet in their direction.

After all that, I must add that we do require a certain amount of vegetable oils; indeed, under some highly unusual circumstances, it would be possible for a person to have a deficiency of these essential fatty acids, but never on this program. So, don't be concerned.

Increasing vegetable fat (oils) is easy. Simply use them in cooking, and when the sodium level is acceptable, use commercial oil dressing on salads. We've also got to strive to get sufficient omega-3 fatty acids from fish as well as the vegetable omega-6. The way to do this is to eat cold-water fish, or to use a judicious level of fish oil supplements.

In Chapter Seven, I pointed out that fish oils, EPA specifically, are important for reducing blood pressure. They do more, however: They significantly reduce the risk of heart disease and inflammatory problems such as arthritis, asthma, and migraine headache. Therefore, I strongly urge you to eat fish—the swimming variety, not shellfish—preferably twice or more each week. If this is not possible, if you truly despise fish, or are allergic (doubtful), then you should use a fish oil supplement of about ½ gram daily. This translates to about three fish oil (not cod liver oil) capsules each day.

There are insidious levels of hidden fat in baked goods, and they are also usually filled with hidden sodium. Baked goods are not compatible with this eating plan. We'll discuss some delicious and healthful dessert alternatives.

Cooking with Fat

Fried foods contain more fat. The bad press of fried foods is the result of fast foods, such as French fries, which are rich in fat and salt and won't work on this program. However, cooking in a wok in small amounts of vegetable oil is an excellent way to maintain the nutritional value of vegetables, fish, and poultry, without adding excessive fat. This eating plan doesn't restrict these foods; you can fry salt free, so go ahead. Many oils are acceptable for wok cooking. The most frequently used oils are peanut, soy, and corn oil. I personally favor olive oil because of its neutrality toward heart disease, but do not let my preference bias your opinion; just be sure to give olive oil a try.

Carbohydrates

Chapter Five introduced the finding that excessive insulin production contributes to high blood pressure by enhancing salt resorption. It follows, from that discussion, that you should not eat foods that will cause high levels of insulin production. You could say that in some people, sugar-rich foods indirectly cause high blood pressure. For our purposes, this means we need to reduce sugar consumption and to seek foods that modulate sugar absorption by slowing its entry into the bloodstream. At the same time, this diet should provide at least 55%, and preferably 60%, of its calories as carbohydrate.

Complex and Simple Carbohydrates

Complex carbohydrates (Chapter Five) are what the word implies: carbohydrates that are more complex than simple sugar. Most carbohydrates consist of either fructose or glucose, two of the most common simple sugars in nature. Fructose is the simple sugar that makes fruits sweet, and it's ubiquitous in naturally sweet foods. Table sugar is a combination of fructose and glucose, named sucrose. Even though it contains both of them, it is still a simple sugar.

The problem with simple sugars is that in the absence of a complex food, like fruit or vegetables, or without a complete meal, they cross the intestinal tract quickly and elevate blood sugar. For example, if you eat candy, or a sweet, sugar-laced soft drink, the surge in your blood sugar causes a surge in insulin output. This surge of elevated insulin, as you know, contributes to sodium retention and elevated blood pressure. The best way to eliminate the problem is to obtain simple carbohydrates from fruit, and the remainder as complex carbohydrates from vegetables, grains, and cereals.

Complex carbohydrates usually consist of glucose, the simple sugar, linked together as a digestible starch. Some starches also contain fructose and other simple sugars, but the major sugar is glucose. The advantage of the complex carbohydrate is that it gets broken down slowly in your digestive system and the glucose enters the bloodstream gradually. To be technical, its absorption is modulated. Modulated absorption of glucose produces a reduced insulin response. And our objective is achieved!

Complex carbohydrates are obtained in natural foods like vegetables, grains, cereals, and their products. For example, excellent carbohydrates are obtained from any vegetable, rice, potatoes, wheat, oats, and also from pasta; so on this program you can eat all the natural vegetables you want. Your only concern is to be sure they are not canned, or prepared with salt, and that your spaghetti sauce is made without salt, using canned tomatoes and tomato paste with no salt added.

A carbohydrate strategy like the one I just described is not difficult to achieve. It means placing emphasis on foods rich in complex carbohydrates and increasing dietary fiber. These dual goals can be achieved by eating lots of vegetables, grains, and fruits. Indeed, for most people, this means shifting toward a more vegetarian emphasis in their diet; usually less meat and processed foods.

This emphasis translates into a breakfast that allows many cereals. For example, it allows oatmeal without salt; shredded wheat; or raisin bran, but excludes all sugared cereals, and cornflakes. If your breakfast centered on eggs and bacon, you can still have the eggs, but no bacon, and you'll still have room for the cereal. The ideal breakfast is cereal with milk and fruit; if you need more, an egg would be okay, unless you can use low-sodium toast.

Lunch should consist of more vegetables, fruit, and grains, if possible. Alternatively, the use of sandwiches causes trouble unless the bread is low in sodium and the sandwich contains generous amounts of lettuce, tomato, avocado, and other vegetables. In Chapter Thirteen, there are several high K Factor sandwiches that are easy to make and taste great! Lunch should be light, and sometimes should contain fish, vegetables, and a salad with low-sodium dressing.

Dinner affords the widest variety of options. Emphasize vegetables, including potatoes, rice, and other high-starch items. Pasta is always good with the correct sauce. Try fruit for dessert. Emphasis should be placed on no salt, lots of starches, and greens, and a low-fat protein food like poultry or fish.

In subsequent chapters we'll cover all the options, but you know the emphasis already. It's on low-salt vegetable foods, with low-fat entrees such as fish and fowl. It also eliminates highly sugared foods and snacks. Obviously, no sugared soft drinks, candy, and sweet rolls. Those items must be eliminated from your food inventory.

Dietary Fiber

Fiber is the undigestible carbohydrate material found in plant foods. It has been called roughage, bulk, crude fiber, and dietary fiber. Although in the strict sense it is not a nutrient because it passes through the system and is not absorbed into the blood, it is one of the most important nutritional components in food. Fiber performs many essential functions on its way through the alimentary canal.

Water is bound to dietary fiber. Some types of fiber, pectin, for example, can bind more than 20 times their weight in water. As a water carrier, fiber increases stool bulk and gives it consistency while maintaining softness. Soft but firm stools are important to regularity and the prevention of a number of intestinal problems like appendicitis, diverticulosis, and hemorrhoids. The added water passing through the intestinal tract helps to dissolve and remove unwanted and sometimes toxic materials. This important function helps to reduce the risk of cancer and other illness. In a previous book, *The Arthritis Relief Diet*, I explained how it reduces flare-ups of arthritis.

Fiber also binds other materials, including simple sugars. This binding causes the sugars to be released slowly as the food materials move down the intestinal tract. This modulation in the release of sugar results in a lower insulin output by the pancreas after a meal that is high in sugar. This modulation of insulin output is essential to your objectives. Fiber does even more; it binds other dietary components such as fat, cholesterol, and even bile acids. All this reduces blood cholesterol. In fact, a high-fiber diet, especially one containing soluble fiber as found in fruits, vegetables, and some grains and cereals, lowers blood cholesterol significantly.

The binding properties of fiber result in diminished constipation, regular bowel movements of soft consistency, modulation of insulin output, and better blood chemistry such as lower cholesterol and triglycerides. People who are not constipated and have regular bowel movements have lower incidences of cancer, heart disease, more moderate blood pressure, and fewer intestinal and bowel problems.

How Much and What Type of Fiber

There are two broad classes of fiber: soluble and insoluble. Within each class of fiber, there are even more subdivisions, so it's not simply a matter of "eat some bran or wheat germ." But it doesn't need to be complicated either.

Variety is the key word to uncomplicate fiber intake—variety in foods of the vegetable kingdom. These include grains, cereals, fruit, and vegetables. If generous servings of each category are eaten regularly, the objective will be achieved. You will know when you have a bowel movement every twenty-four to thirty-six hours; every twenty-four hours is preferable. On average, the stool should be firm, but soft, and light brown in color.

Fiber supplements can be used, if necessary, to increase dietary fiber. Fiber supplements can help a great deal and are easy to use. We'll deal with them in a later chapter.

Water

Water is the second most essential nutrient. We can do without oxygen for only a few minutes and water a few weeks at most. Lack of the next most critical nutrient, the B vitamins, requires months for the first symptoms to develop. In contrast, the symptoms of dehydration can show up in hours.

People require about eight glasses of water daily. Most of us seldom drink that many glasses of water each day. Indeed, we obtain our water in beverages, fruits, and other foods. You should drink more water, and you should be careful of its sodium content. People with high blood pressure should make drinking water a habit, at least four glasses daily. The reason is simply to help facilitate the elimination of sodium. You make the kidneys' work easier.

In addition to drinking more water, you should learn how much sodium is in your water supply. If you live in a hard-water area and have a chemical water softener, you should not drink or cook with the softened water. The reason is that those types of softeners remove calcium salts and replace them with sodium. If that is your situation, either use the hard water for drinking and cooking or purchase bottled water. In contrast to chemical softeners, also called ion exchange systems, are the reverse osmosis and distillation water purifiers. These more costly systems put out soft, very pure water that is excellent for drinking and cooking. Bottled water, especially mineral water, is excellent. Just read the label to be sure it contains very little sodium. Usually bottled water contains less than 1 or 2 milligrams of sodium per glass—that's negligible.

Salt

Americans live in a sea of salt and the islands are made of sugar. Did you know that many, if not most, people get from 7 to 10 grams of salt daily. And many of them never use the salt shaker. How can that be? It's easy. There's an enormous amount of hidden salt in many, if not most, processed and packaged foods. In fact, over 75% of salt intake comes from processed food, as illustrated by the processed foods in Table One. In contrast, nature doesn't work that way. Most natural foods are low in sodium, contain very little chloride, and would be classified as low sodium and low salt. Let's review the differences again.

Low-sodium foods are low in the element sodium. In these foods, usually natural foods, the sodium is in the form of some other salt; for example, sodium acetate, sodium citrate, sodium aspartate, or sodium glutamate to name a few.

Low-salt foods contain little salt, sodium chloride, and they are usually man-made. For example, Nabisco Shredded Wheat contains no added salt, and since wheat happens to be naturally low in sodium, Nabisco Shredded Wheat is both low sodium and low salt. In contrast, Kelloggs All-Bran cereal contains too much sodium for our purposes and most of it is added sodium chloride, common salt. Indeed, Shredded Wheat and All-Bran make a good comparison, since they both start with a natural grain and one company ruins it for our purpose, while the other preserves the natural goodness.

Processors add salt to food for many reasons. It started many years ago when foods were home "canned." Salt was added in those days as a preservative to prevent bacterial growth, and it worked. Botulism, the most dreaded of food-caused illnesses, was often traced to home canning and either not enough salt or not enough boiling in the sterilizer.

As a preservative, salt finds its way into many non-canned foods. This is because it helps to reduce what the food technologists calls "water activity." A food with low water activity usually has very low potential for organisms to grow. Cereal, dried soups, noodle products, gravy mixes, sauce mixes, meat stretchers, and many other dry "packaged" goods are all high-salt examples of the food technologist's art.

But salt came to be added for other reasons; it contributed to taste. For example, some dried soups, like chicken noodle, are 20% salt by weight! And research shows that many people add even more salt to the soup. That means that consumers are getting mostly salt for their money. In fact, the salt in these products costs them about $7 per pound.

Table Two
The Sodium Cost of Processing

I have prepared a table of foods from the vegetable and grain grouping, with some snacks and vegetables. Though this table is not intended to be exhaustive, it illustrates both the amount of sodium and K Factor in natural vs. processed foods. The purpose is for you to get a feeling for the effect that processing has on the food system and the ubiquitous use of salt by the food technologist. The same point is illustrated in Table One for protein rich foods.

This tabulation averages traditional foods to illustrate how processing alters their natural value by increasing the sodium content. These types of processing, in some cases cooking, make them unacceptable for our diet strategy to reduce blood pressure. This tabulation examines the sodium content of a standard serving and the all important K Factor. *Italicized foods are unacceptable on this diet.*

Food	Sodium (mg.)	K Factor
Cereals		
Oats, wheat, barley (cooked without salt)	2	16.0
Cooked with salt as directed	252	0.1
Ready-to-eat Cereal		
High Wheat Bran (Bran Buds, 100% Bran, All Bran)	240	1.2
40% Bran Cereals	262	0.6
Children's Cereals (e.g., Cornflakes, Cheerios, Cap'n Crunch)	290	0.2
Wheat Germ, Shredded Wheat, 100% Natural	6	25.0
Fruits		
Apples, apricots, peaches, pears, etc.	1	over 150.0
Bananas (high potassium)	1	438.0
Fruit canned in syrup	15	over 16.0
Vegetables		
Fresh asparagus, broccoli, string beans	30	over 40.0
Beans, brussels sprouts, corn, etc.		as high as 150.0

Food	Sodium (mg.)	K Factor
The same vegetables		
canned	over 300	0.5
Frozen (no sauce)	same as fresh	
Frozen (with sauce)	same as canned	
Processed Snacks		
Potato Chips	210	1.5
Fritos, tortilla chips, etc.	200	0.2
Pretzels (all types)	450	0.1
Breads		
Wheat flour (whole wheat		
and white)	3	95.0
Oroweat bread (Frozen		
foods some stores)	10	1.0
Low-salt bread (recipe in		
Ch. 14)	2	5.7
Biscuits, including bagels	246	0.15
White bread (slice)	123	0.2
Rye, whole wheat	174	0.3
Crackers	100	0.1
Muffins	200	0.2
Pancakes and waffles		
(most mixes)	200	0.3
Pancakes (recipe in		
Ch. 14)	2	57.0
Beverages		
Coffee (brewed)	2	58.0
Coffee (instant)	1	72.0
Tea (brewed)	19	3.0
Tea (instant)	1	50.0
Soft drinks (club soda,		
colas, etc.)	45	0.1
Juice drinks	less than 20	10 or more
Beer	18	6.0
Wine	about 4	10 or more
Whiskey	1	1.0

Guide to Table Two

Natural foods are low in sodium and high in potassium. Table Two illustrates this point in a number of different ways; it's instructive to consider each of them.

Cereals

Natural cereals are excellent, but as the processing increases, up goes the salt content and down goes the K Factor. One excellent example is oatmeal; cooks up fine without salt, but add the salt and you destroy its value. Ready-to-eat cereals get worse as the processing increases; witness Shredded Wheat, a cereal with very little processing, versus the cereals for children, like Cap'n Crunch. The lesson is obvious. Back to nature!

Fruits and Vegetables

A serving or two of fresh fruit—or even canned fruit— can add potassium to balance other foods that are somewhat higher in sodium. Fruit is excellent for this program as a snack, dessert, ingredient in other dishes, or just about any time. The K Factor of fresh or frozen vegetables (without sauce added) is also excellent. Canned vegetables have lost all their redeeming features. Canned vegetables are so incredibly high in salt that they simply have no place in our program.

Obviously, fresh vegetables and fruits make the best snacks.

Breads

Bread is the staff of life; indeed it is the first thing requested in the Lord's Prayer. However, even though the wheat flour, from which it's made, is low in salt, the end result is not. Oroweat is a fine, low-sodium bread, and there are recipes available for other low-sodium, high-potassium breads.

Beverages

Your coffee or tea break is intact! But don't let yourself become addicted to soft drinks, diet or otherwise. Their sodium content will add up. The best drinks are real fruit juices followed by the fruit juice mixes. Fruit juice is the simplest form of processing; in fact, it only involves squeezing out the juice.

Conclusions from Table Two

Freezing of vegetables and other foods is all right; it does not destroy the value, nor does canning fruit in syrup. Minimal processing of cereals and grains is also acceptable. Most processed foods, however, as we've seen in Table One and Table Two, are simply not acceptable for the person who wants to control high blood pressure by diet.

Obviously, processing contributes an enormous amount of salt to food. Indeed, as illustrated in Table Two, processing completely reverses the natural balance of potassium and sodium. If you are serious about reducing your blood pressure by diet, you will stop eating most processed foods. Develop the ability to read food labels and weed out those unacceptable processed foods.

Reading Food Labels

Food labeling is regulated by the Bureau of Foods of the Food and Drug Administration (the FDA, for short). The FDA requires that every processed, packaged food contain an ingredient declaration. In this ingredient declaration, the components are listed in descending order of content by weight. Therefore, on the ingredient statement, the first component listed is the most abundant and the last is the least abundant. There are a few tricks that are used to make the list look better and often increase profits. For example, rather than use sugar, the processor can use corn syrup (mostly sugar), and high fructose corn syrup, both of which are sugars, but the sweetness is now spread over two ingredients and not one; in fact, actual sugar might not appear until the fourth or fifth ingredient, if at all. With salt, it's not quite that easy, but there are some tricks, such as the listing of water on canned food, so salt moves further down the list.

Nutritional Labeling

Nutritional labeling is mostly voluntary. Voluntary means the manufacturer chooses to give nutritional information. Even if a company does provide nutritional labeling it is not required to put both sodium and potassium on the label, or break down the carbohydrate into sugars, fiber, and complex carbohydrate. But, the nutritional delivery of each serving must be declared.

Nutritional labeling requires the listing of calories, protein, fat, and carbohydrate in grams, and the contribution to the RDA of protein, and seven other nutrients. From this, you can easily evaluate the food with respect to percentage of calories from fat, protein, and carbohydrate. If the manufacturer has included sodium and potassium, you can evaluate its acceptability for this program quickly. Often the manufacturer declares only sodium. Food labeling is most easily illustrated by some examples.

Examples of Ingredient and Nutritional Labeling

Lipton Cup-a-Soup Cream of Chicken Flavor

Ingredients: Nondairy creamer, corn starch, hydrolyzed vegetable protein and other natural flavors, palm oil, dried corn syrup, salt, whey,* monosodium glutamate (natural flavor enhancer), chicken,* guar gum, nonfat dry milk, sodium caseinate, buttermilk,* lactose, onions,* mono- and diglycerides, parsley,* oleoresin turmeric (as color).

This ingredient list is a minefield for a chemist; what is the poor layman to do? I can reduce it to a few simple ingredients for you: Non dairy creamer, starch, oil, corn syrup, flavors, salt, and a group of flavor enhancers.

Nutrition information per serving:

Serving Size	6 fl oz.
Servings Per Container	4
Calories	80
Protein, grams	2
Carbohydrate, grams	9
Fat, grams	5
Sodium, milligrams	840

Percentage of U.S. Recommended Daily Allowances (U.S. RDA):

Protein	2
Niacin	4

Contains Less Than 2% of the U.S. RDA for Vitamin A, Vitamin C, Thiamine, Riboflavin, Calcium and Iron.

You can see that nutrition is not the strong point for this dried soup; in fact, there's precious little nutrition and few calories. But look at the salt content; 840 milligrams of sodium—almost two grams of salt! That's more than a person with high blood pressure should get in two days, let alone in only 80 calories of a beverage.

A person with high blood pressure should not use this product, or any similar product! I don't recommend products with

---

*Dehydrated

this type of formulation for anyone, let alone people with even a hint of elevated blood pressure. Avoid them at all costs.

S & W All Natural Baked Beans

There is no nutritional label on this product; the ingredient list is simplicity itself.

Ingredients: Small white beans with pork in sauce containing water, brown sugar, molasses, salt and mustard.

This product is deceptive, for it implies that the product is natural, and natural white beans would provide only 7 milligrams of sodium and have a K Factor of 6. The salt in the sauce, however, elevates the sodium to at least 800 milligrams and converts the K Factor to about 0.4. Obviously, this product is unacceptable for people who are reducing sodium to control high blood pressure.

Nabisco Spoon Size Shredded Wheat

Ingredients: 100% Natural whole wheat. To help preserve the natural wheat flavor, BHT is added to the packaging material.

Nutrition Information Per Serving:
Serving size ⅔ cup

	Cereal 1 oz.	With ½ cup whole milk
Calories	110	190
Protein	3g.	7g.
Carbohydrate	23g.	29g.
Fat	1g.	5g.
Sodium	less than 10 mg.	60 mg.

[There is other information pertaining to vitamins, minerals and fiber.]

This is an excellent natural cereal for this program. The sodium from milk is less than 60 milligrams and the total is less than the 75 milligrams target for this plan. Since sodium in milk is not in the form of salt, it's all right.

Hungry Jack Extra Lights Pancake and Waffle Mix

Ingredients: Enriched flour [flour, niacin, iron, thiamin mononitrate (vitamin B1), riboflavin (vitamin B2)], yellow corn flour, sugar, baking powder (baking soda) monocalcium phosphate, sodium aluminum phosphate), salt.

Nutritional Label	Mix	Mix Plus Egg, Oil & Milk
Calories	120	210
Protein (g.)	3	6
Carbohydrate (g.)	27	30
Fat (g.)	less than 1	7
Sodium (mg.)	440	490
Potassium (mg.)	105	200

The ingredient list could be simplified to wheat and corn flour, sugar, baking powder, and salt. The manufacturer has added about 800 milligrams of salt, enough to destroy the potassium–sodium ratio and eliminate the product for our consideration. If, however, you wish to make pancakes from scratch, a low-sodium, high-potassium pancake batter is possible.

Putting It All Together

Our brief review of nutrition and the effects of food processing creates a planning challenge for us. On the surface, many of the products mentioned here place salt so far down on the ingredients list as to appear insignificant, but in several examples you see that not only do these foods provide an excess of sodium, but their K Factors are completely unacceptable. Obviously, two things are required. First, a do and don't list will have to become your "bible." Eating out will be a minefield of difficulty, and menu planning is critical if you plan to reduce sodium and salt and improve your potassium intake. Second, you will gain maximum control if you make a decision to use all the information you have available. This means purchasing one or two books on food composition that will guide your purchases and your menu planning.

If this seems a little overwhelming, don't despair; that's why people like me spend their entire career studying the problem and helping people plan their lives. Actual food planning will provide you with incredible variety and sound nutrition, but it does take some work.

I have developed several approaches that will make this task easier.

- Sources of information on food composition that are easy to use and readily available.
- Dietary dos and don'ts and occasionallys. These will identify for you what you can and cannot eat and how to use the "occasionally" concept to indulge yourself and enter the gray areas.
- Plans for eating out. If processed foods are a problem, what about restaurant foods? In restaurants you don't have an ingredient list or a nutritional label, and often, no one can give you knowledgeable answers. I'll show you how to solve this problem.
- Menu planning to see how the plan looks for people who have to eat for low sodium and high potassium, and keep the fat content moderate.

- Recipes for sauces and condiments that will help you eat foods, such as pasta, that are good for you, but require more to make them appropriate.

Additional Reading

The Dictionary of Sodium, Fats, & Cholesterol
Kraus, Barbara
Perigee Publishers, 1983

The Food Book
Stern, Bert, Chilnick, Lawrence D., Sonberg, Lynn
Dell Publishing, 1987

Food Values
Pennington, Jean A.T. & Church, Helen Nichols
Harper & Row, 1985

Chapter Eleven

Potassium-Sodium-Salt

Strategy

Success in controlling high blood pressure without drugs depends upon controlling your sodium intake and the potassium–sodium K Factor ratio. In principle, this task is very simple. The menus in Chapter Thirteen suggest that you can use any completely natural food. Prepare all vegetables by steaming or cooking in oil with no salt; broil or barbecue all meats; broil, poach, or fry fish without salt; and use natural cereals and grains without added salt. All breads must be made from scratch with a salt substitute, or you must use low-sodium breads. Eating out will require great caution, and from time to time, you will either be faced with your own weakness or you may eat something with hidden salt that will upset the balance. There are things that can be done to solve this dilemma; like any journey, let's begin with the first step.

How Much Sodium; How Much Salt?

Sodium-restricted diets are nothing new, and they range from less than 500 milligrams for severe hypertension to an upper limit of 800 milligrams. An 800 milligram sodium diet translates to about 2,000 milligrams of salt. That means at least 5,000 milligrams of potassium would be required to maintain a minimum balance.

Logic dictates that if you include food items that provide more than 75 milligrams of sodium each, and about 250 milligrams for the total meal, you are not going to remain under 800 milligrams of sodium. For example, consider a turkey sandwich on rye bread. The potassium–sodium accounting is as follows:

	Sodium (mg.)	Potassium (mg.)
Bread (2 slices)	348	102
Turkey (2 slices)	32	53
Tomato	1	81
Lettuce (a few leaves)	1	20
Margarine or butter (no salt added)	1	1
	383	237
K Factor (Potassium–Sodium)	0.61	

This sandwich, just about a complete meal, is totally unacceptable on this plan. But if the same sandwich is made with Oroweat low-sodium bread, the accounting changes for the better:

	Sodium (mg.)	Potassium (mg.)
Oroweat low-sodium bread	20	—
Two slices turkey	32	53
Tomato	1	81
Lettuce	1	20
Unsalted butter	1	1
	55	135

Oroweat Bread is available in some areas in the frozen food department. It is not available nationally although other frozen low sodium breads are. Speak to your grocer or health food store manager for assistance. What Oroweat low-sodium bread lacks in flavor can be improved by the use of some spice blends or horseradish; the latter adds about 17 milligrams sodium and 52 milligrams of potassium per tablespoon. Therefore, with a little creativity, a turkey sandwich is not only possible but can be more tasty and even helpful!

K Factor (Potassium–Sodium)		2.5
With horseradish	17	52
	72	187
K Factor (Potassium–Sodium)		2.6

Now let's impose a little California sandwich artistry and add one third of an avocado to the sandwich. This adds excellent texture, great taste, and more potassium.

	Sodium		Potassium
With ⅓ Avocado (see Ch. 15)	7		365
	79		552
K Factor (Potassium–Sodium) With avocado		7.0	

Many other interesting alternatives are possible, including a high K Factor bread, but the point should be clear. By using low-sodium bread, horseradish, and avocado, you have created an excellent low-sodium–high-potassium meal. add an apple and a cup of coffee or tea, and the meal is complete and great!

Natural Foods

With very few exceptions, nature has taken care of our task. Natural foods contain much more potassium than sodium by a large margin. Natural foods have another bonus; they are low in both sodium and salt. Therefore, if you can go strictly by nature, you almost don't need to read any further.

High-Potassium Foods

Some foods are naturally very high in potassium, in addition to being low in sodium. These foods can often serve as snacks, and can be added to other foods or eaten with them to help the balance. For example, two thirds cup of raisins provides 750 milligrams of potassium and only 12 of sodium. So, as a snack, added to cereal, or in ice cream (already okay), raisins boost the K Factor significantly. The same is true for dried figs and dates. I'll list these foods in the "dos" so you can get into the habit of selecting snacks and condiments that are not only risk free but also contribute to your K factor.

Low-Sodium Foods

Supermarkets have some low-sodium foods available, and more are appearing all the time. You can help increase these sections and these foods by voting with money. You vote every time you purchase them, because money is what counts with the manufacturer and the supermarket owner. The more the products sell, the greater variety and flavors you will find and the more shelf space will be devoted to low-sodium foods.

Low-sodium salad dressings are an outstanding example of the good food technologist's capability. For example, most brands of Russian or Thousand Island salad dressing provides about 125 to 130 milligrams of sodium per tablespoon (and who only uses a tablespoon?) and very little potassium, so their K factor is nil. In contrast, the low-sodium (and usually low-calorie) salad dressings contain only 2 milligrams sodium and 32 of potassium, giving them a K Factor of 16. From earlier discussions, I know you are aware that salads are excellent for this plan. They naturally provide high potassium, low sodium, and no salt. So, by using one of these salad dressings, you actually make the salad better and don't sacrifice flavor.

Other low-sodium foods, especially prepared foods like soup, seem bland. This is because we are accustomed to more salt and the materials available to the technologist often leave no other option. They can be spiced up, however. For example, a single drop of Tabasco adds only 2.5 milligrams of salt (an insignificant amount), and six drops can make a low-sodium soup taste much better, at a cost of only 15 milligrams of sodium. Another approach is to use a tablespoon of horseradish for taste. Horseradish adds 17 milligrams of sodium and 52 milligrams of potassium, improves the K Factor, and adds a modest amount of texture.

Salt Substitutes

In general, the best salt substitutes are not made from potassium chloride. Remember, sodium retention is really salt retention and if you get sodium from one source and chloride from another, the nephrons in your kidneys must deal with it as sodium chloride. It's like added salt to them. Therefore, you must read the label carefully and select products made from other potassium salts. Potassium gluconate and potassium bitartrate are the most common.

Salt substitutes can improve a meal with their potassium content. There are times when it serves as more than a flavor enhancer in cooking and is necessary to the recipe, such as in low-sodium bread. In addition, other people eating with you will want to add it to their food for taste.

Salt substitutes are excellent for those occasions but should be used only when necessary.

Salt substitutes are good for cooking, but not essential, and there are reasons to be cautious about consuming excess potassium. While 5,000 to 10,000 milligrams of potassium (5 to 10 grams) should be fine, it is possible by excessive use of salt substitutes to exceed that level. More than 10 grams of potassium is excessive, so use caution with salt substitute, and emphasize spices and herbs instead.

Sauces and Gravies

Most commercial sauces and gravies are not acceptable on this plan. They are prepared with far too much salt and there is no room for compromise. That is why the recipe section is short; it emphasizes low-sodium preparation of sauces. There are some available that provide taste without salt listed in the next chapter. There is, however, a natural alternative: Use garlic, onions, shallots, spices, and other herbs. For example, a little garlic sautéed in olive oil on a barbecued or broiled steak, on hamburger, fish, or poultry provides an excellent eating sensation. Try grated ginger over fish, poultry, and salads, or sautéed with other foods to accomplish the same objective—good taste and good health.

Summary

The guidelines are clear: Minimize sodium and increase potassium naturally. Use natural foods to increase potassium and balance any food that increased sodium intake and worked against the potassium–sodium K Factor ratio. Salt substitutes can help a little, but they are by no means the answer, you've got to take care in selecting the best ones. Low-sodium foods can be excellent and go a long way to make life more pleasant. Seek them out whenever possible and use natural condiments to improve their flavor.

Additional Reading

For recipes and spices that eliminate sodium and do not require the use of salt substitutes, write to:

The American Spice Trade Association
580 Sylvan Avenue
Englewood Cliffs, NJ 07632

Chapter Twelve

Food at Last

This chapter follows a sequence you might recognize as breakfast, lunch, dinner, snack foods, desserts, and beverages. Most foods are listed by sodium and potassium content, and the K Factor. With this information, you can plan your menus accordingly.

Objective: Sodium–Potassium

Your objective is to reduce daily sodium intake to 800 milligrams or less; preferably about 500 milligrams. In recalcitrant high blood pressure, 500 milligrams is often the upper limit. The same foods that will help you dramatically reduce your sodium will help elevate your potassium to more than 4,000 milligrams. In summary, you want to finish each day with a K Factor of 3 or more, and with a total sodium intake of 800 milligrams or less. In Chapter Eleven, I said that the upper limit of acceptable sodium content, in a single food serving of about 3.5 ounces should be 75 milligrams. If the food is especially rich in potassium, and sodium is less than 100 milligrams it can be used, but make those foods the exception.

Food Tables: Dos and Don'ts

The following tables will help you select foods that will give you a new lease on life. The data on these foods are from several sources, books that I have listed in the last section of this chapter. Serving size is a problem whenever food is discussed. Serving size is usually expressed as 3.5 ounces (100 grams) or in other terms, like a single piece of fruit or other convenient serving.

Cooked Cereals

<u>Do</u>

Cooked cereals are excellent if no salt is added in their preparation. Instant cooked cereals (add hot water) are often unacceptable because salt is used in the processing. Serving Size: One ounce. Milk is not included in these servings. It is tabulated separately. Each cup of milk adds 122 milligrams sodium and 377 milligrams potassium.

Cereal	Sodium (mg.)	Potassium (mg.)	K Factor
Barley	1 to 4	45 to 127	45
Corn grits, regular	0	54	54
Maypo	6	158	26
Oats	1	99	99
Ralston	3	115	38
Roman Meal	2	227	113
Whole Wheat	1	129	129
Wheatena	4	140	35
Cream of Wheat	2	33	16

Don't

Following the recipe on the box and adding salt destroys
cooked cereal for this plan. These cereals taste excellent
without added salt. If your taste buds crave salt, add six
drops of Tabasco per serving. I know it sounds strange in
cereal, but Tabasco only adds 2.5 mg. sodium. Six drops, a
lot, adds only 15 mg. and the taste is fine. Another alternative: Don't even use milk; try your cereal with apricot
nectar. It tastes great, reduces sodium, and elevates potassium even more.

Ready-to-eat Cereals
Do

Serving Size: One ounce. Milk is not included in these
analyses. Milk is tabulated separately. A cup of milk usually adds 122 milligrams sodium and 377 milligrams potassium to each serving. See milk tabulation where low sodium
is expressed, however.

Cereal	Sodium (mg.)	Potassium (mg.)	K Factor
Frosted Mini Wheats	8	97	12
Granola Nature Valley	3	142	47
Puffed Rice	0	10	10
Puffed Wheat	1	50	50
Quaker 100% Natural	12	140	12
with Raisins	12	139	12
with Apples	14	140	10
Shredded Wheat and			
Shredded Wheat 'N Fiber	3	102	34
Super Sugar Crisp	25	105	4
Wheat germ, toasted	1	268	268

Occasionally

These cereals, in my opinion, are borderline because they are moderate in sodium and not high in potassium. Consequently, they have a poor K Factor. The addition of milk elevates the sodium content very close to the 200-milligram cutoff, even though the K Factor is acceptable. Therefore, only use them occasionally and remember to eat other low-sodium, high-potassium foods in compensation.

Cereal	Sodium (mg.)	Potassium (mg.)	K Factor
C. W. Post with Raisins	49	58	1.2
Heartland Natural	72	95	1.3
Heartland with Coconut	57	104	1.8
Heartland with Raisins	58	107	1.8

Don't

Most ready-to-eat cereals cannot be used on this plan. I have identified those that can be served. You can recognize those that cannot by a simple test; they usually have sodium on the nutritional label.

Milk for Cereal and Beverage

Do

All milks, canned, dry, condensed, and whole, are "do" for beverages or for cereals. The sodium in milk is not in the form of sodium chloride (salt) and, while it is higher than desirable, it is acceptable; note that low-sodium milk can be obtained. I strongly recommend avoiding high-fat milk and using the low-fat varieties. This tabulation summarizes the pertinent information.

Milk (one cup)	Sodium (mg.)	Potassium (mg.)	K Factor
Low-fat (1% fat)	123	381	3.0
Low-fat (2% fat)	122	377	3.0
Skim	126	406	3.2
Whole (3.5% fat)	122	351	2.9
Low-sodium whole	6	617	102.0
Skim dry (reconstituted)	161	538	3.3
Whole dry (reconstituted)	119	426	3.6

Beverage Mixes for Milk

Although people following this plan are expected to be adults, some of us never outgrow our desire for flavored milk. These milk mixes are fine, but be sure to add the sodium and potassium from the milk to the total figures.

Mix	Sodium (mg.)	Potassium (mg.)	K Factor
Chocolate powder	54	168	3.0
Hershey Chocolate Powder	36	89	2.5
Quick Strawberry Powder	81	206	2.5

Eggs

Do

In general, eggs are acceptable because the sodium is not in the form of sodium chloride and their protein quality is excellent. When we get into menu planning, you will see that a breakfast of half a cantaloupe, fried egg, and cereal is fine in moderation.

Eggs	Sodium (mg.)	Potassium (mg.)	K Factor
Eggs (one large)	69	65	0.95
Egg, fried or omelet	144	58	0.40

Don't

Eggs are usually acceptable on this eating plan, but the methods of preparation usually cause trouble. If you fry, don't add salt to the oil. Omelets should be made with a few drops of Tabasco or horseradish in place of salt. They should always be vegetarian, with ingredients such as onions, mushrooms, and tomatoes, for example.

Breads
Do

Oroweat bread is the most readily available low-sodium bread. It is purchased in the frozen section, thaws quickly, can be used for toast or for sandwiches. The sodium content is insignificant.

Bread (2 slices)	Sodium (mg.)	Potassium (mg.)	K Factor
Oroweat	10	NA	NA
Recipes (Ch. 14)	2	114	57

Don't

Breads and baked goods account for much of the hidden 5 to 10 grams of salt that Americans consume daily. If you like sandwiches and want to beat high blood pressure, you must learn to like Oroweat or other low-sodium bread. Remember that not all grocers carry Oroweat bread and there are others available; usually in the frozen section. Be sure to ask.

Fruits
Do

Fruit toppings for cereals and fruit as an accompaniment to any meal, especially breakfast, is excellent. Fruit is not only acceptable, it is highly recommended. You can't eat too much fruit, nor can you eat too many varieties. In this tabulation, I have selected the average; for example, I have tabulated "apples" and "bananas." Please recognize that there are many varieties and I have summarized the average value.

Fruit	Sodium (mg.)	Potassium (mg.)	K Factor
Apples, medium (with skin)	1	159	159
Applesauce, canned (3½ oz. unsweetened)	2	91	45
Apricots, raw, 3 medium	1	313	313
Canned (average)	3	139	46
Banana, medium	1	451	451
Blackberries, ½ cup (similar for canned and frozen)	0	141	141
Blueberries, 1 cup	9	129	14

Fruit	Sodium (mg.)	Potassium (mg.)	K Factor
Boysenberries, 1 cup, canned	2	207	104
Cantaloupe, 1 cup pieces	14	494	35
Cherries, 10 sweet	0	152	152
Cherries, 1 cup sour, canned	9	119	13
Dates, 10 dried	2	541	270
Figs (1 medium)	1	116	116
Fruit cocktail, ½ cup, canned	4	118	29
Grapefruit, ½ medium	0	158	158
Grapes, 1 cup	2	176	88
Honeydew melon, ¼ small	12	251	21
Kiwi fruit, 1 medium	4	252	63
Lemon or lime, 1 medium	1	80	80
Mango, 1 medium	4	322	81
Nectarine, 1 medium	0	288	288
Orange, 1 medium	1	250	250
Papaya, medium	8	780	98
Peach, medium	0	171	171
Canned, 1 cup	11	317	29
Pear, medium	1	208	208
Pineapple, 1 cup	1	175	175
Plum, medium	0	113	113
Prunes, 10	3	626	209
Raisins, ⅔ cup	12	746	62
Raspberries, 1 cup	0	187	187
Strawberries, 1 cup	2	247	123
Tangerines, medium	1	132	132

Fruit Juices

Do

Fruit juices, like fruit, are generally low in sodium and rich in potassium. They can be used to offset a meal component that is not rich in potassium but is low in sodium. For example, a poached egg on Oroweat toast and a glass of apple juice are balanced in sodium and potassium, even though the egg itself is not. Except where noted, serving size is 8 ounces.

Fruit Juice	Sodium (mg.)	Potassium (mg.)	K Factor
Apple juice	7	296	42
Apricot nectar	9	286	32
Cranberry juice	10	61	6
Grape juice	7	334	48
Grapefruit juice	2	400	200
Lemon or lime juice (1 T)	0	19	19
Orange juice	2	496	298
Papaya nectar	14	78	6
Peach nectar	17	101	6
Pineapple juice	2	334	167
Prune juice	11	706	64
Tangerine juice	2	440	220
Tomato juice or V-8 Juice (low sodium)	47	550	12

Don't

Any fresh fruit and fresh fruit juice is excellent on this plan. Therefore, the only don'ts are sugary juice drinks, processed by man, that contain only a small amount of real juice. Fruit is not canned or frozen with salt, so it is usually fine; similarly for fruit juice. You can't use too much of either category.

Meat

Most non-organ meats are fine for people on this plan. In Chapter Ten, I tabulated the "caloric cost" of protein, illustrating that white meat is less caloric than red. To help you reduce the fat content and consequently your caloric intake, I have included the percentage of calories from fat in this section. I have done this for beef, pork, and white meat. And appropriately, I have broken it into low-, medium-, and high-fat selections, listing the high-fat meat as "occasionally." Low-fat meat, in general, is excellent on this diet. It is low in sodium, rich in potassium, and if lean cuts are selected with excess fat trimmed, its caloric content is fine for this program.

Preparation of meat, including poultry, is important. It should always be broiled or barbecued with sauces, or salt. Condiments such as garlic, onions, shallots, ginger, and other herbs, spices, and appropriate vegetables, add flavor and zest to meat without increasing either its fat or sodium content. In all these tabulations, the serving size is the conventional 3½ ounces.

Do

Beef Low Fat

These cuts provide less than 25% of their calories as fat.

Beef Cut	Sodium (mg.)	Potassium (mg.)	K Factor
Hamburger (lean)	41	480	11
Shank (lean)	60	370	6
Top round	46	547	12

Do

Beef Medium Fat

These cuts of beef provide 25% to 40% of their calories as fat. They are acceptable on a weight-controlled program.

Beef Cut	Sodium (mg.)	Potassium (mg.)	K Factor
Chuck (selected lean)	60	370	6
Club steak (lean only)	27	236	9
Flank steak	67	344	5
Porterhouse (lean only)	26	232	9
Rib roast (lean only)	17	169	10
Bottom round	51	552	11
Pot roast (lean only)	18	152	8
Sirloin (lean only)	34	349	10

Occasionally

Beef High Fat

These cuts of beef are fine for control of high blood pressure, but due to their fat content they are recommended only occasionally and never on a weight-loss diet.

Beef Cut	Sodium (mg.)	Potassium (mg.)	K Factor
Chuck	60	370	6
Hamburger (medium fat)	40	382	9
Rib roast (lean and marbled)	57	438	8
Rib eye steak	60	370	6

Beef Cut	Sodium (mg.)	Potassium (mg.)	K Factor
Pot roast (lean and marbled)	43	309	7
Sirloin (lean and marbled)	57	545	9
Roast or ground			
T-bone	49	378	7
Tenderloin	30	288	9

<u>Do</u>

Lamb Medium Fat

These cuts of lamb provide 26% to 40% of calories as fat.

Cut	Sodium (mg.)	Potassium (mg.)	K Factor
Arm chop (lean only)	49	286	6
Leg (marbled)	82	492	6
Leg (lean only)	52	312	6
Rib chop (lean)	43	252	6

<u>Occasionally</u>

Lamb High Fat

These cuts of lamb provide over 40% of their calories as fat.

Cut	Sodium (mg.)	Potassium (mg.)	K Factor
Arm chop (marbled)	66	388	6
Blade chop (lean)	46	276	6
Loin chop (marbled)	37	218	6
Rib chop (marbled)	68	398	6

Do

Pork Medium Fat

These cuts of pork are moderate in fat—that is, 26% to 40% of their calories are from fat.

Cut	Sodium (mg.)	Potassium (mg.)	K Factor
Blade (lean)	44	311	7
Butt (lean)	29	209	7
Ham fresh (lean)	54	382	7
Loin chop (lean)	41	386	9

Occasionally

Pork High Fat

These cuts of pork are high in fat. Over 41% of their calories are derived from fat.

Cut	Sodium (mg.)	Potassium (mg.)	K Factor
Blade (marbled)	78	551	7
Ham fresh (marbled)	61	434	7
Loin chop (marbled)	52	500	10
Tenderloin (lean)	55	509	9

Do

Veal

These cuts of veal are low to moderate in fat content; less than 34% of their calories are derived from fat.

Cut	Sodium (mg.)	Potassium (mg.)	K Factor
Arm steak (lean)	46	452	10
Loin chop (lean)	47	342	7
Rib chop (lean)	35	329	9
Sirloin (marbled)	38	342	9
Sirloin (lean only)	38	342	9

Occasionally

Veal High Fat

These cuts of veal are high in their fat content and over 40% of their calories are derived from fat.

Cut	Sodium (mg.)	Potassium (mg.)	K Factor
Arm steak (marbled)	51	503	10
Chuck (medium fat)	80	500	6
Cutlet	54	527	10
Loin chop	54	384	7
Rib roast	80	500	6
Rib chop	41	387	9

Occasionally

Organ Meats

In general, organ meats are excessive in fat, but I have selected these because they are moderate in fat. Some organ meats are so high in sodium, that even though it is not always sodium chloride, it is often excessive for our purposes.

Organ	Sodium (mg.)	Potassium (mg.)	K Factor
Hog heart	65	128	2.0
Calves' liver (raw)	73	281	4.0
Hog liver (raw)	73	261	3.6
Lamb liver (raw)	52	202	4.0

Don't

Meats

Processed meat, whether beef, veal, or lamb, is simply unacceptable. This includes the prepared list. Since these foods are unacceptable. I have not included sodium, potassium, or the K Factor ratio.

Don't Beef

> Breakfast strips
> Beef burgundy
> Frozen and canned sliced beef
> Frozen or canned chipped beef (several brands)
> Corned beef
> Frozen meatloaf
> Frozen or canned salisbury steak

Don't Pork

> Bacon bits
> Canadian bacon
> Cured bacon
> Cured ham
> Ham loaf
> Ham steaks
> Sweet and sour pork
> Sausages

Don't Veal

> Frozen Veal Parmigiana

Don't
Luncheon Meats, Franks, Spreads

There are virtually no processed meats that can be eaten by people following this plan to control high blood pressure. This includes chicken and turkey ersatz meats such as turkey pastrami, bologna, and franks.

Barbecue loaf
Sausage (including bockwurst, blood, bratwurst, Polish
    luncheon, smoked and turkey)
Corned beef loaf
Frankfurter
Processed ham (including loaf, etc.)
Bologna of all types
Mortadella
Loaves (olive, mother's, pepper, pickle, picnic)
Salami of all types
Sandwich spreads (including Spam)
Thuringer
Turkey ham, turkey loaf, pastrami
Vienna sausage

Poultry

In general, poultry is excellent for any dietary program. If it is roasted, broiled, or barbecued without skin, or the skin is removed after cooking, it is low in fat and excellent in sodium and potassium, but even poultry can be high in fat if not selected correctly.

Do
Chicken

Cut	Low-Fat Chicken Sodium (mg.)	Potassium (mg.)	K Factor
Breast, roasted (without skin)	63	220	3.5
Drumstick, roasted (without skin)	42	108	2.5

Cut	Sodium (mg.)	Potassium (mg.)	K Factor
Medium-Fat Chicken			
Breast (with skin)	69	240	3.5
Drumstick (with skin)	47	119	2.5
High-Fat Chicken			
Wing, roasted	25	57	2.0

Do
Turkey

Cut	Sodium (mg.)	Potassium (mg.)	K Factor
Low-Fat Turkey			
Light meat, roasted (without skin)	64	305	
Medium-Fat Turkey			
Light meat (with skin)	63	285	4.5
Dark meat (with skin)	76	274	3.6
Dark meat (without skin)	79	290	3.7
Ground turkey	74	260	3.5
Wing	74	130	1.7

Do

Cut	Sodium (mg.)	Potassium (mg.)	K Factor
Other Low-Fat Poultry			
Pheasant (without skin)	37	262	7.0

Cut	Sodium (mg.)	Potassium (mg.)	K Factor
Other High-Fat Poultry			
Duck (with skin)	59	204	3.5
Duck (without skin)	65	252	3.9
Goose (with skin)	70	329	4.7
Goose (without skin)	76	388	5.0

Don't
Processed Poultry

Remember, I listed turkey bologna, pastrami, etc., as don'ts under luncheon meats. These are unacceptable. It is that simple!

Fish

In general, fish contain fat that is polyunsaturated, and many fish are low in fat. There is a sodium concern, however, because many fish contain over 75 milligrams in a normal serving. While this is a caution, it is a minor caution, since the sodium is usually not in the form of sodium chloride (salt). Therefore, select fish at least two or three times weekly, and use shellfish in moderation.

Fish is best when simply baked, broiled, or poached. If you fry it, do so without added salt and in olive oil. For zest and flavor, use spices such as ground ginger, bay seasoning, and others. Use onions, garlic, shallots, and other condiments to enhance the flavor of the fish. A few drops of Tabasco is excellent.

Do

Type	Sodium (mg.)	Potassium (mg.)	K Factor
Abalone	70	250	3.6
Sea bass	68	256	3.8
Bluefish	74	250	3.4
Carp	50	286	6.0
Codfish	105	386	3.8
Croaker	87	234	2.7
Flounder	56	366	6.5
Haddock	61	304	5.0
Halibut	54	449	8.0
Herring	74	420	6.0
Kingfish	83	250	3.0
Lingcod	59	433	7.0
Lobster	60	265	4.0
Mackerel	68	256	4.0
Mullet	81	292	3.6
Perch	79	269	3.4
Pompano	47	191	4.0
Red snapper	67	323	5.0
Salmon	45	399	9.0
Squid	47	191	4.0
Swordfish	56	366	6.0
Tuna	40	293	7.0
Sea trout	75	317	4.0

Occasionally
Shellfish

Shellfish must be eaten with caution in this dietary program. Although they are low in fat, they are often high in sodium. The exceptions are soft clams and oysters. One serving of shellfish could use 25% of the daily allowance of

800 milligrams of sodium. Therefore, menu planning is absolutely critical when these fish are used.

Type	Sodium (mg.)	Potassium (mg.)	K Factor
Clam (soft)	36	235	6.0
Clam (hard)	205	311	1.5
Mussels	289	315	1.0
Oysters	73	121	1.6
Scallops	255	396	1.6
Shrimp	140	220	1.6

Don't

Don't use processed, breaded, or batter-dipped fish, especially fish fillets. This list does not include sodium and potassium content because these foods are too high in sodium to be acceptable under any circumstances. If you can find any that are low sodium, use them.

Type
Crab cakes, deviled crab, crab imperial
Canned crab
Batter, breaded, country-seasoned fish fillets or other pieces
Fish sticks, breaded and frozen
Fillet almondine
Lobster Newburg
Lobster paste
Canned or frozen oysters, clams, or mussels
Canned fish, or fish packed in brine, unless specified "low sodium"
Sardines in any sauce
Shrimp, breaded, paste, or French fried

Vegetables

Do

Fresh vegetables and fresh frozen vegetables are excellent for this program. They are naturally high in potassium and low in sodium. Do not use frozen mixed vegetables, however, unless they are on the "do" list of prepared mixed frozen vegetables. And, never, under any circumstances, should you use canned vegetables.

Vegetables can be prepared in a variety of ways, ranging from boiling to frying in a wok with small amounts of oil. None of these methods will change their sodium–potassium content. However, when cooking rice, or any vegetables, never add salt. If salt is called for, as it usually is in cooking rice, for example, it is optional and can be cooked without it. If necessary, in cooking, olive oil will serve the same purpose.

Vegetable	Sodium (mg.)	Potassium (mg.)	K Factor
Artichoke, 1	30	301	10
Asparagus	1	183	183
Avocado	21	1,097	52
Bamboo shoots	20	709	35
Beans, not canned	7	416	59
Beets, 2 medium	60	335	6
Black-eyed peas	1	303	303
Broccoli, 1 large fresh or frozen	10	267	27
Brussels sprouts, fresh or frozen	10	273	27
Cabbage, raw	20	233	10
Carrots, 1 large	47	341	7
Cauliflower	13	295	23
Celery, 1 stalk	63	170	3

Vegetable	Sodium (mg.)	Potassium (mg).	K Factor
Chilies, red	9	420	47
Collard greens	43	401	9
Corn, white, frozen	4	226	56
Corn, yellow, fresh	11	219	20
Cow peas	8	229	29
Cucumber	3	80	27
Eggplant	2	214	107
Green beans, fresh or frozen	2	136	68
Kidney beans, fresh	3	340	113
Lentils	3	249	83
Lettuce	9	264	29
Lima beans, fresh or frozen	75	478	6
Mung bean spouts	5	223	45
Mushrooms	15	414	27
Mustard greens	32	377	12
Okra	2	174	87
Onions	10	157	16
Parsley	45	727	16
Peas	2	316	158
Pepper, 1 bell	13	213	16
Potato, 1 medium	3	407	136
Radish	18	322	18
Rhubarb	2	148	74
Rice, cooked without salt	1	42	42
Scallions, 5 medium	5	231	47
Spinach, raw	71	470	7
Squash, average	2	250	125
Sweet potato	22	540	24
Tomato, 1 large	6	488	81
Turnip greens, frozen	12	184	15

Do
Frozen Mixed Vegetables

All serving sizes are declared on box or are the standard 3½ ounces.

Vegetables	Sodium (mg.)	Potassium (mg.)	K Factor
Broccoli, carrots, & water chestnuts	22	247	11
Broccoli, cauliflower, & red peppers	18	203	18
Broccoli, corn, & red peppers	11	199	18
Carrots, peas, & onions	53	147	3
Cauliflower, green beans, & corn	9	166	18
Green beans, corn, carrots, & onions	10	163	16
Peas, carrots, & onions	60	158	3

Snacks

"Snack" is a word that is too often synonymous with highly salted or highly sugared foods eaten between meals. It conjures up chips, fries, things smothered in cheese, etc. Snacks can be apples and vegetables, such as carrot sticks. These snacks, with their excellent potassium content, actually have a beneficial effect on your high blood pressure. This listing contains snacks that can be acceptable if done without salt.

Do

These snacks are acceptable for this program and can be used effectively. The serving size is expressed so you can gain insight into how much you can use.

Type	Sodium (mg.)	Potassium (mg.)	K Factor
Popcorn (1 cup without added salt)	—	28	28
Potato chips (1 oz. Lay's with no salt added)	4	380	95
Dried Fruit			
Raisins (⅔ cup)	12	746	62
Figs (10)	1	85	85
Dates (10)	2	541	270
Dried apricots (10 halves)	3	482	160
Nuts			
Almonds, unsalted	1	104	104
Almonds, salted (1 oz.)	55	216	4
Brazil nuts (⅓ cup)	1	670	670
Cashews, unsalted, roasted (20–26)	8	232	29
Chestnuts (½ cup)	2	410	205
Peanuts, roasted, unsalted (1 oz.)	1	200	200
Pecans (12 halves)	1	63	63
Seeds			
Sunflower seeds	8	258	33

Don't

All other processed snacks are unacceptable unless you can purchase snacks that have no sodium added and provide less than about 25 milligrams sodium in a normal serving.

Beverages

Do

Life without beverages would be like days without sunshine. Indeed, the "coffee break," which includes beverages from coffee to Perrier water, is an international tradition. And, alcoholic beverages are part of a way of life for man people. Therefore, I have compiled a list that preserves the coffee break and cocktail hour, and slakes the thirst.

Beverage	Sodium (mg.)	Potassium (mg.)	K Factor
Alcoholic Beverages			
Beer (12 oz.)	18	115	6
Liquor (1 oz.)	1	1	1
Whiskey, gin, rum, vodka (1 oz.)	0	1	1
Wine (3½ oz.)	10	116	11
Coffee, Tea, Cereal Beverages (6 oz.)			
Cereal coffee (Postum)	3	97	33
Coffee, brewed	2	117	50
Instant coffee	1	72	72
Flavored coffees (average)	25	250	10
Tea (regular)	19	58	3
Tea (instant)	1	50	50
Iced tea from mix (sweetened)	13	94	7

Occasionally (Rarely)
Carbonated Beverages

Many carbonated beverages contain more than 75 milligrams of sodium, with insufficient potassium to redeem them. Therefore, they do not appear on this list. In contrast, some beverages do appear because their sodium content is low enough that their overall contribution is insignificant if used in moderation and if the diet is correct. Twelve-ounce servings.

Beverage	Sodium (mg.)	Potassium (mg.)	K Factor
Coca-Cola	14	—	—
Cola	20	7	0.3
Ginger Ale	30	5	0.2
Flavored Soda	less than 40	about 8	0.2
Seven-Up	4	0	—
Tonic water	2	1	0.5
Diet Coke	33	—	—
Diet Rite	37	1	0.03
Diet Sprite	45	—	—
Pepsi Light	42	12	0.3
Tab	27	—	—
Mineral water	less than 5	usually trace	—

Desserts

Desserts are often an important part of the meal, and dairy products provide an excellent opportunity for eating pleasure without penalty. Whenever possible, whether you're eating ice cream or sherbet, top with any fresh fruit. The fruit not only provides variety and eating pleasure but also contributes potassium without a sodium penalty.

Serving size of bulk ice cream is one cup.

Do
Dairy Desserts

Dessert	Sodium (mg.)	Potassium (mg.)	K Factor
Chocolate ice cream	75	240	3
French custard	84	241	3
Creamsicle	27	82	3
Fudgsicle	55	173	3
Ice cream bar (chocolate coating)	28	107	4
Chocolate ice milk	61	175	3
Dryer's Grand Light ice cream (all flavors)	50	about 175	3

Cream and Whipped Toppings

For some people cream is essential in coffee, on fruit, or as whipped cream or whipped cream substitute. The products on this list can effectively convert fruit from another low-sodium dessert to a great dessert. You gain the low sodium and high potassium of fruit with the taste and texture of whipped cream.

Topping (1 Tablespoon)	Sodium (mg.)	Potassium (mg.)	K Factor
Cream, including half and half, light to heavy, including whipped	6	19	3
Sour cream	12	29	3
Whipped toppings (either Cool Whip or powdered mixes)	3	6	2

Puddings and Gelatin Desserts

Some of these desserts are borderline, but if served with fruit, or whipped topping, the sodium–potassium K Factor ratio is acceptable. Some, like gelatin desserts, are fine, especially when fruit is added to the mix or served as a topping. Your store may carry another brand. If so it probably has a composition similar to the ones shown here.

All servings one cup.

Dessert	Sodium (mg.)	Potassium (mg.)	K Factor
Chocolate pudding, homemade	81	246	3
D-Zerta chocolate	82	227	3
Rice pineapple	15	55	3
Gelatin desserts	8	180	22

Dessert Toppings

These toppings can be served on gelatin, ice cream, pudding, or with fruit.

Serving size is three tablespoons.

Topping	Sodium (mg.)	Potassium (mg.)	K Factor
Cherry topping	17	380	22
Chocolate fudge	32	60	2
Chocolate syrup (Hershey)	20	48	2
Pecans in syrup	—	125	125
Pineapple	17	28	2
Walnuts in syrup	—	88	88

Occasionally
Candy

I do not advocate the use of candy. It is something we can do without, and we never use it in our family. However, in recognition of people's frailties and that sometimes it seems socially necessary, and the possibility that you may want to give a gift to a high-blood-pressured friend, this list is presented. Remember our discussions about excessive insulin!

Type	Sodium (mg.)	Potassium (mg.)	K Factor
Individual Candy			
Chocolate Kisses (6)	25	115	5
Chocolate-covered almonds	17	153	9
Chocolate-covered brazil nuts	13	153	12
Chocolate with cream center	2	30	15
Gumdrops (28)	10	1	0.1
Hard candy (6)	9	1	0.1
Lifesavers	3	—	—
Malted Milk Balls	28	113	4
Candy Bars			
Hershey Dark Chocolate	1	97	97
Nestle Crunch	50	110	2
Hershey Golden Almond	17	140	8
Kit Kat	28	96	3
Hershey Krackel	49	116	2
Hershey Milk Chocolate	26	119	5
Mr. Goodbar	16	162	10

Low-Sodium Salad Dressings and Condiments
Do

Low-sodium products are excellent for this plan. Other condiments such as Tabasco sauce can also be used to make plain, low-sodium food taste much better.

Product	Sodium (mg.)	Potassium (mg.)	K Factor
Horseradish	17	52	3.0
Homemade sour cream sauce	7	13	2.0
Tabasco sauce (1 teaspoon)	22	3	0.1
Tabasco (6 drops)	15	1	0.1
Perc for natural spices (see note at end of chapter)	1.5	22	14.6
Low Sodium Salad Dressings			
Russian	2	33	16
Thousand Island	2	33	16
Vinegar	2	5	2

Low-Sodium Soups
Do

Low-sodium soups by Campbell generally taste bland and seem watery, but they can be made much better with the addition of 4 to 6 drops of Tabasco or a tablespoon of horseradish.

Low-sodium onion soup, tomato, or cream of mushroom are all excellent if made more tasty as above.

Canned and Dry Soups
Don't

Canned soups, even Campbell's "Special Menu," are
unacceptable. Dry soups are even worse. For example, a
serving of many soups provides over one gram of sodium,
all in the form of sodium chloride. I have not listed these
products because they are simply too high in sodium and
their potassium content is even worse. Do not be coerced
by the statement "no salt added," or "homemade." The
sodium content is excessive.

Mustard and Ketchup

Neither of these condiments is acceptable on this program. Learn to use other flavorings.

	Sodium (mg.)	Potassium (mg.)	K Factor
tomato ketchup	156	54	0.3
mustard	188	20	0.1

Salt Substitutes

An ideal salt substitute is made from only potassium
gluconate or potassium bitartrate! These are organic salts
formed between potassium and a derivative of the sugar,
glucose, or tartaric acid. In very technical terms, for you
chemists, the salt formed from potassium hydroxide and
gluconic or tartaric acid to make potassium gluconate or
tartrate. Do not use a salt substitute that consists only of
potassium chloride. Most salt substitutes will contain some
potassium chloride, but consist primarily of other potas-

sium salts. I urge you to purchase the Perc products described below and at the end of the chapter since they avoid the use of salt substitutes completely and eliminate the problem of chloride.

Spices, Herbs, and Flavorings
Do

For thousands of years, spices and herbs were used to enhance the flavor of foods. Spices have a rich history; they were also used to protect food from spoiling and to cover bad food with exotic flavor. We are no longer faced with problems of contaminated or spoiled food. In fact, we can now use herbs, spices, and condiments strictly for pleasure. In this strategy they go much further and help us to achieve a strategy of food without salt and rich in potassium. All amounts are one teaspoon.

Food	Sodium (mg.)	Potassium (mg.)	K Factor
Ground Spices Dried			
Allspice, basil, bay leaves, chervil, cinnamon, clove, garlic, ginger, mace, marjoram, mustard, nutmeg, oregano, pepper, rosemary, sage, savory, tarragon, thyme, turmeric	Trace	Average 30	30
Seed Spices			
Anise, caraway, celery, coriander, cumin, dill, fennel, fenugreek, mustard, poppy	1	20	20

Food	Sodium (mg.)	Potassium (mg.)	K Factor
Powdered Spices			
Chili pepper, curry, garlic, ginger, cinnamon, mustard, paprika, parsley, pumpkin pie spice	1	20	20
Perc from natural spices (see note at end of chapter)	1.5	22	14.6

Don't

You cannot use flavored salts. These are mostly salt and are flavored with other materials. They include, among other, the following: Lemon and Pepper Seasoning, Salt and Spice, Buttersalt™, Onion Salt™, Celery Salt™, Salt Seasoning, Salad Supreme™.

Oils

Do
Cooking Oils

Cooking oil (frying or wok) should not be excessive in PUFA because there is good reason to believe changes take place from the heat of frying that can be detrimental to health. With both that and the need to prevent heart disease in mind, I have prepared a list of oils that I recommend in descending order of quality. You can obtain their content from the table in Chapter Seven.

Olive oil
Peanut oil

Sesame oil
Shortening
Soft margarine
Butter

Do
Oils for Dressing

In making salad dressings and wherever oil is required in non-frying cooking, I recommend the light high-PUFA oils. I have prepared the following list in descending order of quality.

Safflower oil
Sunflower oil
Corn oil
Soybean oil
Olive oil
Peanut oil

Do
Exotic Oils

Some gourmet stores provide oils from nuts that are especially rich in the omega-3 fatty acids that, in your body, produce EPA. These include walnut oil, almond oil, and others. They are expensive, but if you can afford to, use them.

Supplements

I strongly recommend a food supplement that provides about half the RDA for all the vitamins and minerals, except calcium and vitamin C. I treat calcium differently because whether you get enough or not depends upon how much milk or dairy products you consume.

Basic Supplement

A general supplement should provide the following in one tablet.

Vitamin Nutrient	Content	% RDA
Vitamin A	2,500 I.U.*	50
Vitamin D	200 I.U.*	50
Vitamin E	15 I.U.*	50
Vitamin C	30 mg.	50
Folic Acid	0.2 mg.	50
Thiamin (B-1)	0.75 mg.	50
Riboflavin (B-2)	0.86 mg.	50
Niacin	10 mg.	50
Vitamin B-6	1 mg.	50
Vitamin B-12	3 micrograms	50
Biotin	0.15 mg.	50
Pantothenic acid	5 mg.	50

*International Units

Mineral Nutrient	Content	% RDA
Calcium *	0.5 grams	50
Phosphorus*	0.4 grams	40
Iodine	75 micrograms	50
Iron	9 mg.	50
Magnesium *	200 mg.	50
Copper	1 mg.	50
Zinc	1 mg.	50
Selenium	50 micrograms	50

*Most multivitamin-multimineral supplements will not contain this much calcium, phosphorous, and magnesium. You probably will require a separate supplement for these minerals.

You will not usually be able to purchase a supplement that provides the complement of nutrients I recommend. If you can, I recommend that you take that much each day, preferably at breakfast. Chances are, though, that the supplement you find in the store will not have that profile. Most general supplements provide the RDA for all nutrients except calcium, magnesium, and phosphorus. If that is the case for your supplement, I recommend you take a calcium magnesium supplement and don't worry about phosphorous. You will get more than enough phosphorus in your diet, so there is no cause for concern.

How Much Calcium and Magnesium?

If you do not drink milk or use any other dairy products, I urge that you get a total of 800 milligrams of calcium and 200 milligrams of magnesium from supplements daily. This can be accomplished by selecting a calcium magnesium supplement. The supplement will probably contain about 200 to 300 milligrams of calcium and about 50 milligrams of magnesium. Simply take two or three of them; one with each meal is an excellent plan.

EPA/Fish Oil Supplements

If you do not eat fish, I recommend that you strive for about 500 milligrams of EPA daily. Since EPA or fish oil capsules usually contain 180 milligrams per capsule, you should take three of them.

Vitamin C

Controversy around this vitamin will continue into the next century: I hope it will be settled for my great-grandchildren by the twenty-second century. I believe many people require more than the 65 milligrams RDA for this vitamin. I base my belief on research and comments that indicate that the needs of our immune system are more demanding than we realize. Also, I believe that the stress of modern life forces more demands on vitamin C in its role as a cancer preventive. So, I believe that the RDA should be about 250 milligrams and therefore I recommend that we eat lots of fruit, fruit juice, and vegetables, and take supplemental vitamin C. In fact, 500 milligrams daily is not, in my opinion, excessive. And many very healthy experts on the subject take more than that.

Beta Carotene

In recent years it's become clear that some nutrients help prevent cancer. Beta carotene, a nutrient that our bodies convert to vitamin A as it is required, has a function in its own right—to protect against environmental cancer. If you follow this plan, your diet will be rich in beta carotene because it's obtained from vegetables. If you want added insurance, however, I recommend that you use 10,000 I.U. daily.

Fiber Supplements

Many fiber supplements are available. They are usually packaged as a powder that requires you to put a tablespoon in an eight-ounce glass of water and drink it down. Most of them are a semisoluble fiber from psyllium seeds and are very effective. My only caution is that you evaluate their sodium content. It is essential that they do not contain more than about 10 milligrams of sodium per serving and that they have a K Factor of 3 or more.

Additional Reading

If you only needed to know sodium content, there are a number of food tabulations available that are adequate, but to succeed on this program, you need to find out sodium and potassium levels. That is limiting, but there is one excellent source book available.

Food Values of Portions Commonly Used, 14th ed. by Jean A. T. Pennington, Ph.D., R. D., and Helen N. Church, B.S., Harper and Row, 1985.

Two other books, which do not list potassium content:

The Food Book, produced by Bert Stern, Dell, 1987.
Perc™ Salt Free Spices

Tone Brothers is a company that has provided spices since 1873 (they're solid). They provide excellent seasonings for many types of food, but they provide even more—toll-free salt-exchange telephone numbers. Call:

1-800-247-7515 or, in Iowa, 1-800-372-6071
Or write to:
Tone Bros., Inc.
Box AA
Des Moines, IA 50301

Chapter Thirteen

Menus:
One Day at a Time

Blood pressure control without drugs is an ongoing objective that begins now with your next meal, or your next snack. I have planned some menus for you that illustrate just how easy eating for low sodium and high potassium can be.

Breakfast

My mother always says that each day should begin with a good breakfast. She's right! Reasons for a good breakfast begin with the need for the correct kind of nourishment and extend to deeply rooted habits; you feel better having started the day out right. Morning nourishment should consist of protein, complex carbohydrate, fiber, and up to one third of the daily nutrient requirements. This translates to many options, and I'll try to explore enough to show you how it's done.

Basic Breakfast

This is my breakfast; it's simple and very effective. It consists of hot cereal, usually oatmeal (cooked without salt) with raisins, sweetened with maple syrup, accompanied by either one half a grapefruit or a one quarter of a melon, and followed by two cups of tea. If you review this breakfast, you will see that it is very healthy, contains ample protein, the excellent fiber of oatmeal, and fruit, along with sufficient carbohydrate.

Food	Sodium (mg.)	Potassium (mg.)	K Factor
Melon, ¼	14	494	35
Oatmeal	1	99	99
with raisins	3	186	62
Maple syrup, 2 tablespoons	4	70	17
Milk, 1 cup	123	381	3
Tea, 2 cups	38	114	3
Totals	183	1,344	7.3

The K Factor for this entire meal is 7.3.

In this section I have listed seven breakfasts that are filling, varied, and good to eat. They provide a choice of foods that illustrates the variations possible on this plan. Not one contains 200 milligrams of sodium, and all have a K Factor of over 5. And they do not exhaust all the possibilities from the dos and don't lists.

Breakfast One

	Sodium (mg.)	Potassium (mg.)	K Factor
Grapefruit, ½	0	158	158
Oatmeal (no salt)	1	99	99
Milk on oatmeal	123	381	3
Raisins in oatmeal, ⅙ cup	3	186	62
Tea, 2 cups	38	114	3
Totals	165	938	5.7

Breakfast Two

	Sodium (mg.)	Potassium (mg.)	K Factor
Orange juice, 1 glass	9	281	31
Cantaloupe, ¼	14	494	35
Nabisco Shredded Wheat	3	102	34
Milk, 1 cup	123	381	3
Coffee, two cups	4	234	58
Totals	153	1,492	9.7

Breakfast Three

	Sodium (mg.)	Potassium (mg.)	K Factor
Orange Juice, 1 glass	9	281	31
Grapefruit, ½	0	158	158
Mushroom omelet			
Eggs, 2	138	130	0.9
Mushrooms, 1 cup	15	414	28
Coffee, 1 cup	2	117	58
Totals	164	1,100	6.7

This omelet can be seasoned with horseradish or with 3 or 4 drops of Tabasco sauce.

Breakfast Four

	Sodium (mg.)	Potassium (mg.)	K Factor
Scala Müsli Oatmeal			
(Chapter 14)	1	99	99
with apricot nectar	9	286	32
Oroweat toast	10	10	1
with marmalade,			
1 tablespoon	4	9	2
Coffee (brewed)	2	117	
Totals	**126**	**521**	**20**

Breakfast Five

	Sodium (mg.)	Potassium (mg.)	K Factor
French Toast (Two slices)			
Oroweat, or other low-			
sodium bread, dipped			
in batter of:	10	10	1
Egg	69	65	1
Milk, ½ cup	61	190	3
Nutmeg ½ teaspoon		10	20
Maple syrup,			
5 tablespoons	10	176	17
Orange juice, 1 glass	2	474	237
Totals	**152**	**925**	**6.1**

Breakfast Six

	Sodium (mg.)	Potassium (mg.)	K Factor
Quaker Natural Cereal	12	140	12
with sliced Banana	1	451	451
Milk, 1 cup	123	381	3
Grapefruit juice, 1 glass	2	400	200
Coffee, 1 cup	2	117	58
Totals	**140**	**1,488**	**10.6**

Breakfast Seven

	Sodium (mg.)	Potassium (mg.)	K Factor
Steak 3½ ounces	60	370	6
One egg, over easy	69	65	1
Honeydew melon, ¼	12	251	21
Coffee, 2 cups brewed	4	234	58
Totals	**145**	**920**	**6.3**

I don't advocate this "lumberjack" breakfast, but it makes the point that even a big breakfast can be eaten as long as it's balanced.

Lunch

Traditionally, this meal comes at the middle of one's daily activity. Even people who work at night, in the reverse of the day world, have a "lunch" hour. The size of this meal varies throughout the world; in some countries it is light and quick; in others, heavy and long. Not surprisingly, in our country, indeed, our continent, it is a light meal on the average, but for many, lunch is the setting for business discussions. This "business" lunch doesn't stop with traditional people of commerce meeting in restaurants; it includes the beautiful people who make society work. I'm thinking of the countless numbers of women and men who volunteer their time, most often lunch time, usually hosted in their homes, for local arts, sports, school services, health services, and other things that when woven together make up the cultural fabric of our society.

Despite its social or business purpose, lunch must meet the standards I have established. The objective remains firm; an upper limit of about 200 milligrams of sodium for the complete meal, no single item over about 75 milligrams of sodium, with a desired K Factor of 3 or more. These standards are easily met by anyone preparing lunch at home, even if it is going to be eaten from a lunch box 50 stories above the ground. The difficulty comes for those who must, for many reasons, eat at restaurants. So, I have divided luncheon into two approaches: first those where you are in charge of food preparation and, in a later section, where you are selecting from a menu. In the former, I can provide interesting menus; in the latter, I have provided guidelines and examples.

Lunch Sandwiches

Being an incurable sandwich eater, I empathize with the problem of having a good sandwich for lunch. Sympathizing with the plight of sandwich eaters everywhere, I have recognized two basics; in Chapter Fourteen you will find three bread recipes that produce excellent breads including white bread (traditional), whole wheat (wholesome), and pita bread (delicious); there's also an excellent mayonnaise that tastes like the real thing. For example, if you like pita bread and eat a sandwich daily, the recipe in Chapter Fourteen will make 20 pitas that keep well. That's twenty very tasty sandwiches; it's not as much extra work as it appears. You can also use commercial low-sodium breads that, for all practical purposes, provide very little sodium and little potassium. What they do provide is the basic structure to hold the sandwich contents together.

Sliced Turkey Sandwich

This sandwich is prepared from turkey breast that is cooked and packaged or sliced turkey from the deli. Do not confuse it with the turkey sold as "turkey loaf" that is prepared in brine and loaded with sodium. The turkey I recommend is "natural" and has only been roasted. You can also do it yourself by simply roasting a turkey and removing the skin.

Item	Sodium (mg.)	Potassium (mg.)	K Factor
Low-sodium bread	10	10	1
Turkey, 2 large slices	64	305	5
Unsalted butter,			
1 tablespoon	1	1	1
Horseradish, 1 tablespoon	17	52	3
Totals	92	368	4

Sliced Turkey Potassium Powerhouse

I call this my potassium powerhouse because it's a sandwich that would do well in any restaurant and it's a powerhouse of nutrition. Its variations are obvious, permitting use of many seasonings and spices.

Item	Sodium (mg.)	Potassium (mg.)	K Factor
Bread, (for example, pita, Ch. 14)	2	114	57
Turkey, 2 slices	64	305	5
Avocado, ⅓	7	366	52
Onion, 2 slices	2	32	16
Mayonnaise (Ch. 14), 1 tablespoon	7	88	13
Totals	82	905	11

Sliced Roast Beef

To many people the word "sandwich" means "beef." I hope they will change their ways and learn to enjoy turkey, chicken, fish, and vegetarian sandwiches.

Item	Sodium (mg.)	Potassium (mg.)	K Factor
Bread, 2 slices (Ch. 14)	2	114	57
Roast beef, 2 slices	38	400	10
Tomato, 2 slices	1	90	—
Horseradish, 1 tablespoon	17	52	—
Lettuce, 2 or 3 leaves	—	—	—
Totals	58	656	11
Made with commercial low-sodium bread	76	560	7

The difference in sodium, potassium, and the K Factor gives you an idea of why it is worthwhile to make your own bread.

Tuna Fish Sandwich

A tuna sandwich is as American as apple pie. New Yorkers alone consume 594 million tuna sandwiches annually! Miami is the poorest tuna sandwich city (per capita) in the U.S. at 106 million annually. Therefore, it would be unpatriotic of me not to provide a tuna sandwich recipe.

You *absolutely* must choose *low-sodium* tuna canned in water! No substitutes! One acceptable alternative is to cook your own tuna, separate it from the bones, break it into flakes with a fork, and use it as the basic tuna for a sandwich. I assume that you are using homemade low-sodium bread.

Item	Sodium (mg.)	Potassium (mg.)	K Factor
Bread, 2 slices (Ch. 14)	2	114	57
Tuna, 2 ounces (⅓ can low sodium)	24	159	7
Mayonnaise, 2 tablespoons (Ch. 14)	14	176	13
Lemon juice	0	19	—
Chopped celery, ½ cup	63	171	2.7
Totals	103	639	6

This is not the most ideal tuna sandwich for this plan, so I made a better tuna sandwich using a very ripe avocado. A very ripe avocado is obtained by purchasing an avocado and allowing it to stand at room temperature until it is soft to the touch. The complete recipe for this sandwich with its many options is in Chapter Fourteen, but the salient features follow:

Tuna Avocado Powerhouse

Item	Sodium (mg.)	Potassium (mg.)	K Factor
One pita pocket (Ch. 14)	2	114	57
Tuna, 2 oz. low sodium	24	159	7
Avocado, ⅓ per sandwich	7	365	52
Tomato, ¼	1	46	46
Onion, 1 slice, chopped	1	16	16
Parsley, chopped	2	17	8
Totals	37	717	19

Sandwich Accompaniments

The sandwiches I have described make an excellent entree for a good high-blood-pressure-beating lunch. But the following accompaniments to a sandwich can make a good luncheon great. By selecting a suitable beverage, soup, salad, or fruit, you can enhance your eating pleasure with good nutrition.

Basic Green Salad

A salad made from lettuce, tomatoes, avocado, peppers, and other high K Factor salad ingredients is good for you and excellent for this eating plan. The moderate salad I've created consists of tomato, lettuce, green and red peppers, chopped parsley, cucumber, and chopped scallions. As long as the salad you make does not use canned beans or other vegetables, it will be fine. What about salad dressing?

Nature has solved the problem very effectively by making common cider vinegar and olive oil low-sodium food components. Add spices and herbs, and it has a high K Factor. Chapter Fourteen contains an excellent low-sodium oil-and-vinegar recipe flavored with spices that goes with any salad. Alternatively, you can use commercial low-sodium dressings or make your own from recipe books. See how the salad complements a sandwich.

Item	Sodium (mg.)	Potassium (mg.)	K Factor
Tomato, ½	2	183	92
Lettuce, ¼ head	9	175	19
Green pepper, ½	7	107	15
Red pepper, ½	7	107	15
Parsley, 1 tablespoon	4	73	18
Cucumber, ⅓	3	80	26
Scallions, 5 chopped	5	232	46
Oil and vinegar dressing (Ch. 14)	—	15	—
Totals	37	972	26

Soup

Canned soups, except for the few bland-tasting low-sodium varieties, were ruled out in Chapter Ten because they contain too much sodium. The low-sodium soups may be flavored with Tabasco sauce, horseradish, and other spices, or a low-sodium high–K Factor soup must be made from scratch. Chapter Fourteen guides you to cookbooks that provide a wide variety of hot and cold soups low in sodium and rich in potassium.

I have selected an American standby, cream of tomato soup, to illustrate the effective use of a recipe. This soup can be prepared, saved by refrigeration, and served later. It can be taken to work in a thermos.

Soup	Sodium (mg.)	Potassium (mg.)	K Factor
Cream of tomato (See recipe in Ch. 14)	16	1,200	74

This soup, accompanying any of the sandwiches presented in this section, would make for an excellent lunch. But more, the lunch would be under the 200 milligrams of sodium limit and would provide an outstanding K Factor. Suppose we evaluate our sandwich-salad or sandwich-soup lunches. Recognize that these are illustrations, but they indicate that with a little effort, an excellent lunch is easily achievable.

Sandwich-Soup and Sandwich-Salad Scoreboard: Some Examples

Luncheon	Sodium (mg.)	Potassium (mg.)	K Factor
Basic turkey sandwich	92	368	4
Salad	37	972	26
Coffee, 1 cup	2	117	58
Totals	131	1,457	11
Turkey Powerhouse	82	905	11
Salad	37	972	26
Coffee, 1 cup	2	117	58
Totals	121	1,994	16
Tuna Powerhouse	37	717	19
Basic tomato soup	126	1,200	74
Coffee, 1 cup	2	117	58
Totals	55	2,034	37

Luncheon	Sodium (mg.)	Potassium (mg.)	K Factor
Roast beef	76	560	7
Salad	37	972	26
Coffee, 1 cup	2	117	58
Totals	115	1,649	14

If these lunches are combined with the sensible breakfasts suggested, you will be through two major meals with less than 350 milligrams of sodium and an excellent level of over 2,000 milligrams potassium (some combinations are close to 3,000 milligrams), all with one meal to go.

Lunch Salads

Preparation of lunch salads usually relies on the use of mayonnaise; the recipe in Chapter Fourteen solves that challenge. For example, a chicken, tuna, shrimp, or crabmeat salad served on lettuce, avocado, tomato, or green pepper is an excellent lunch main dish. In addition, many other approaches to salads can be taken. The rules are simple.

• Any fresh fruits or vegetables can be used without limit.
• Chicken, turkey, pheasant, or fresh seafood can be used generously.
• Canned tuna can be used if the water-packed, low-sodium variety is selected.
• Mayonnaise or other dressing requires a special recipe. A basic mayonnaise recipe is provided in Chapter Fourteen, but additional dressings can be found in the cookbooks recommended.

Other Home-Cooked Lunch Menus

Chapter Twelve identifies a broad range of dos and don'ts for eating pleasure. Since your dietary program restricts sodium and urges high potassium, your menus are only bounded by your imagination, your pocketbook, and your interest in cooking. I urge you to use natural foods prepared from scratch. Some foods that are especially nutritious but receive little emphasis follow.

Beans

Beans, often maligned with the term "musical fruit," are especially rich in protein—the dietary fiber that helps reduce cholesterol—and they are low in fat. Their nourishment value is beyond question. Preparation is the only challenge, because you cannot use canned beans. So why not learn to make them from scratch? Beans can be used in an endless variety of recipes, so long as you omit salt and use an appropriate salt substitute. Once you have begun to prepare beans from scratch, you can make chili, bean soup, bean salads, a number of Mexican dishes, and you can use beans as an ingredient in soups. Beans and rice can be flavored in an endless variety of ways, making a nourishing meal that is low in fat and sodium and is an excellent source of protein and dietary fiber.

Pasta

Spaghetti is an excellent food for this program. In addition to its fine K Factor, it provides protein with little fat and excellent carbohydrate. But pasta is only as good as its sauce. Chapter Fourteen contains a recipe for a spaghetti sauce with meat options, made with low-sodium foods and fresh tomatoes. A clam sauce, similarly designed, is also provided.

A pasta lunch is excellent on this program. This basic spaghetti sauce contains spices, but can be further enhanced with a salt substitute.

Item	Sodium (mg.)	Potassium (mg.)	K Factor
Spaghetti (2 ounces dry)	1	115	115
Sauce	8	681	85
Totals	**9**	**796**	**88**
With meat	15	93	6
Totals	**24**	**889**	**37**
With clams	36	235	5
Totals	**45**	**1,031**	**23**

Served with a salad, this is an excellent luncheon or dinner.

Spanish Rice

Spanish rice prepared with tomatoes, beans, mushrooms, and other vegetables (as in Chapter Fourteen), is low in calories, a good source of protein, and has a high K Factor. This ethnic dish lends itself to many variations using meat, seafood, and an almost endless variety of vegetables.

Item	Sodium (mg.)	Potassium (mg.)	K Factor
Basic Spanish Rice	19	688	36

Obviously, the variations on some of the basic luncheons are endless. Once you have purchased a good cookbook and are willing to use a little imagination, the delicious menu varieties available to you are boundless. Most of them require very little use of salt substitutes, but do make use of a variety of spices that help introduce even more taste and variations.

Fruit

Fruit should always accompany your lunch. You need the excellent fiber it provides (with no fat) and its superb K Factor. Ideally, fruit will be taken in its raw form, for example, as an apple, pear, or orange. A slice of melon or a dish of mixed fruit is excellent. And as Chapter Twelve indicates, if berries are your choice, they can be enhanced with whipped cream or whipped cream substitute.

Fruit affords a number of natural benefits. It's naturally sweet, and complemented with fiber. It modulates the entry of natural sugars into the bloodstream. But more, it provides the satiety that comes with bulk and the satisfaction of munching. Its vitamins and minerals are good. Fruit has everything going in its favor. The old saying "An apple a day keeps the doctor away" is as timely now as it's ever been.

Dinner

I have treated dinner in two ways: first, as the traditional meal, prepared at home, eaten by the entire family, even if the family is just a husband and wife; second, as a meal often eaten out. Eating in restaurants requires planning and a willingness to ask questions. I offer some guidelines and specific dos and don'ts for eating lunch and dinner out later in this chapter.

No matter what has transpired during the day, dinner should emphasize low-fat entrees with the exception of some fish, such as salmon. Dinner should also contribute to daily fiber consumption and it should be rich in complex carbohydrates, not sugar. If this sounds familiar, it is. As always, emphasis should be placed on low-fat, high-complex-carbohydrate foods with a high K Factor. This translates as fish, poultry, lean meat, vegetables, grains (including pasta), and fruit. The boundaries of high blood pressure allow just about any natural food, but we can optimize by selecting judiciously.

An Ideal Home-Cooked Dinner: Dinner One

This is a dinner we serve in our house two times each week. It emphasizes fish as the entree and fresh vegetables with rice as the major complex carbohydrate source. The Key lime pie is a personal favorite and requires no more work than many desserts that people serve; however, any number of desserts can be substituted. An excellent accompaniment for this dinner would be a glass of Chardonnay. Tea, with its moderate caffeine, would be a fine after dinner beverage.

Following our sample breakfasts and lunches, this dinner would complete the day with a sodium level well below 800 milligrams and a K Factor substantially above 3. All without Spartan living, I might add!

Item	Sodium (mg.)	Potassium (mg.)	K Factor
Salmon, broiled	64	306	5
Asparagus	1	183	183
Long-grained rice	1	105	105
Salad with dressing (see lunch)	37	972	26
Key lime pie (Ch. 14)	49	149	3
Totals	152	1,715	11

Dinner Two

Another typical dinner at our home is one cooked in a wok or large skillet. I have cooked it in ten minutes on television shows. In designing this dinner, I have included a Chinese dish (chicken) with an Italian starch (pasta) and an American dessert (carrot cake). Surprisingly, the components enhance one another very well and the experience is delightful. Gourmet flare is possible within our boundaries. The dinner would be enhanced by a glass of slightly robust white wine such as Riesling. And dessert could be followed by coffee or tea. In keeping with the tradition of the entree, green tea would be appropriate.

Item	Sodium (mg.)	Potassium (mg.)	K Factor
Chicken with broccoli and cashews (Ch. 14)	78	676	9
Served over angel hair pasta (also can be served with rice)	1	115	115
Carrot cake	46	376	8
Totals	125	1,167	9

Dinner Three

As a boy, I thought linguine was mined, not made from wheat. All kidding aside, the accompanying clam sauce (Chapter Fourteen) is made from readily available items and is delicious. The serving size is moderate; however, it would not be excessive if doubled. In true Italian tradition, it is served with a large salad, dish of broccoli, and a dessert of fruit. Contrary to tradition, it should be served with a rich red wine.

Item	Sodium (mg.)	Potassium (mg.)	K Factor
Linguine and white clam sauce (Ch. 14)	52	524	10
Salad	37	972	26
Broccoli	15	382	25
Melon for dessert	53	484	9
Red wine	10	116	12
Totals	167	2,478	15

Dinner Four

To avoid offending my non-Italian friends, it is essential to serve an American classic. This dinner is served best as a weekend afternoon dinner. It surprises many people on this dietary program just how acceptable it can be. The problem of rolls or bread must be faced head on by baking them according to a salt-free cookbook.

Item	Sodium (mg.)	Potassium (mg.)	K Factor
Rib roast (juice used for gravy—Ch. 14)	80	500	6
Baked potato	6	755	126
Sour cream on potato	12	34	3
Lima beans	2	675	377
Butter, unsalted on beans	2	2	1
Salad	37	972	26
Rolls (homemade— Ch. 14)	2	114	57
Red wine, 1 glass	10	116	12
Apple pie (Ch. 14)	12	307	26
Light ice cream on pie	50	175	4
Totals	133	3,534	27

Obviously this gargantuan American classic meets our standards. I even chose a traditional dessert. This meal is large! If prepared as I have described it, this meal is very low in sodium. It is not a meal for someone with heart disease or who is overweight, but the ubiquitous nature of this dinner option illustrates the versatility of our dietary program.

Dinner Five

Baked stuffed trout is low in fat and is an excellent choice of fish, one that receives compliments even from people who do not enjoy fish. Trout is generally available in supermarkets. It is one of the few freshwater fishes that is harvested, iced, and transported to the supermarket in a day or two, in contrast to saltwater fish, which are often over several weeks old before being sold.

Baked stuffed trout is an excellent dinner for anyone on a weight-reducing diet. If you're not dieting, add a light white wine and the carrot cake dessert. From the sodium–potassium accounting, there is easily room for the wine or another beverage.

Item	Sodium (mg.)	Potassium (mg.)	K Factor
Baked stuffed trout (Ch. 14)	69	922	13
Broccoli, steamed	15	382	25
Brown rice (Ch. 14)	18	131	7
Carrot cake	46	376	8
Totals	148	1,811	12

Dinner Six

Pork chops are an American standby. Pork is not excessive in calories if the fat is properly trimmed. This recipe makes generous use of fruit and spices. I have selected a traditional menu of green beans, potato, a small salad, and a light chiffon pie for dessert.

Although the pork chop is somewhat high in sodium and a few pie ingredients are elevated in sodium, this dinner comes in well below the upper limit of 200 milligrams of sodium, and its K Factor is excellent. It illustrates more of the variety available on a low-sodium diet.

Item	Sodium (mg.)	Potassium (mg.)	K Factor
Pork chop (Ch. 14)	75	949	13
Green beans	2	136	68
New potatoes	3	407	135
Small salad	37	972	26
Lemon chiffon pie	39	112	3
Wine, one glass (optional)	10	116	12
Totals	166	2,692	16

Dinner Seven

Fillet of sole West Indies is an excellent example of the use of fruit in a fish recipe. This meal can be easily prepared in about 30 minutes and is nice for a summer evening. I have selected a gazpacho as a prelude, with rice for carbohydrate, and a simple green salad. We have served this meal often with compliments from everyone. No one would think for one moment that this meal has special dietary applications.

Item	Sodium (mg.)	Potassium (mg.)	K Factor
Gazpacho (Ch. 14)	13	412	32
Fillet of Sole (Ch. 14)	100	1,069	11
Rice	1	42	42
Green salad	37	972	26
Strawberry mousse (Ch. 14)	17	58	3
Totals	187	2,776	15

Conclusions

These meal menus can all be mixed and matched. They illustrate the ease of achieving a low-sodium diet with adequate potassium intake from readily available food. It is definitely within everyone's grasp to maintain a sodium intake below 500 milligrams and obtain more than sufficient potassium.

Dining Out for Lunch and Dinner

My rule of thumb for dining out at any time is "eat natural." And, that's not easy in most restaurants, unless you apply the dos and don'ts already identified. Let me go through some generally foolproof rules.

- Broiled fish, meat, and fowl with no sauce in natural juices is usually safe. If you explain to the waiter that you are following a strict low-sodium diet, he will work with you.
- Sautéed vegetables are generally safe so long as you emphasize the "low sodium" because many chefs "salt" the frying pan. It prevents the hot oil from spattering. For example, sautéed mushrooms or other vegetables are usually all right.

- Steamed vegetables such as broccoli or asparagus are safe. Query about a sauce. Explain that you can't eat the sauce and if they insist, put it on the side.
- Potatoes and pasta without a sauce are usually the best complex carbohydrates. Rice is out; restaurants always add salt to rice so forget it. Stick to potatoes and pasta with garlic, olive oil, and spices, or no sauce at all. Use a little olive oil, garlic, and lemon. Purchase the Perc™ seasonings and always carry them with you (Chapter Thirteen).
- Appetizers are difficult because they usually rely on sauce, but that reduces your selection to shrimp with horseradish, not cocktail sauce. Smoked salmon or trout with plain horseradish is generally safe. An alternative is to request either a small salad (oil and vinegar) or mushrooms sautéed without salt. Avocado or artichoke is also fine without the sauce. Artichokes go well with oil and vinegar and avocados can be eaten without any sauce.
- Dessert is actually much easier than most people are willing to recognize—eat fruit. It would be a rare restaurant indeed that did not have a piece of fresh fruit or some berries. They make a fine dessert, and a little whipped cream or artificial whipped cream is okay. But you can take a risk and enjoy a fruit mousse, or fruit pie without the crust. That's correct: The salt is in the crust; and fruit part might be somewhat caloric, but it's usually low in sodium.
- Restaurant bread and rolls are not for us. They simply cannot be eaten because of their salt content. You can learn to get along without them; you'll be thinner for doing so and your blood pressure will be lower.

Eating Out Guidelines

While basic menus are easy to prepare at home once you've got the hang of it, eating out is not the same.

Restaurants often serve meals prepared and frozen in central kitchens, salt gets added to many items, and sauces often come from institutional-size cans. In general, the amount of sodium and potassium in restaurant food is simply not known. But you can wade through the uncharted minefields of restaurants and cafeteria food without your own personal dietician. All you've got to do is prepare a list of dos and don'ts and questions to ask as you survey your choices. You'll be able to maintain your health and not emerge as a person everyone wants to avoid.

DON'TS

DON'T eat bread or rolls, not even one slice.

DON'T eat cheese, cheese sauces, or cheese on any foods, including salad.

DON'T order sauces or gravy on any foods, don't order foods requiring sauce.

DON'T order foods fried in a batter, such as breaded veal, squid, chicken, or fish.

DON'T order fried foods unless they are simply fried in oil with no salt added either before or after.

DON'T order pies, cakes, chiffons, mousse, or puddings for dessert.

DON'T use enhancers such Worcestershire sauce or A-1 sauce.

DON'T eat rice in restaurants; it's always salted.

DON'T eat soup in restaurants.

DOS

DO order fish, chicken, meat broiled without breading. This includes hamburgers (no cheese) without extenders.

DO eat chicken without skin and *do not* use any sauces.

DO eat steamed, boiled, or even fried vegetables if they are not canned and salt is not added in cooking.

DO always eat a salad and two fresh vegetables with lunch. An excellent selection is an ungarnished baked potato. You can enhance it with sour cream, unsalted (sweet) butter, or unsalted margarine. A better approach is to use lemon juice.

DO use avocado for an appetizer or get an artichoke and eat it with oil and vinegar.

DO use vinegar and oil on your salad; no substitutes.

DO eat fresh or canned fruit for dessert, if fresh is not available.

Questions To Ask

You must learn to ask questions in a restaurant. Don't ever be intimidated; it's your body and your health and they'll be handing you the check. Most chefs do not mind the extra request of broiled fish or chicken with no salt. And, if things need spicing, ask for Tabasco sauce; remember, a few drops go a long way.

ASK May I have the salad with oil and vinegar on the side?

ASK Can my vegetables be prepared without salt?

ASK May I have some unsalted French fries?

ASK Will you make my salad without cheese?

ASK Can the chef fry or sauté my fish, or mushrooms, and so on without using salt or monosodium glutamate?

ASK May I have a plain hamburger on the plate without fries, if they are salted?

ASK Do you have any fresh fruit for dessert?

By asking these questions, following the dos and don'ts, and remembering that natural foods are all right, you're "home free" as the saying goes.

What To Drink?

Alcohol must be seriously limited (Chapter Six). The goal is to drink sociably but not excessively. It is best not to take an alcoholic beverage at noon, but if you must, wine spritzers (wine with soda) are good because they make a little wine go a long way. I strongly urge you to restrict yourself to the equivalent of one glass of wine daily. That translates to a glass of wine, one mixed drink, or a can of beer. The best approach is to learn control and decide what meal is enhanced best by the glass of wine.

The best drinks are mineral water with a twist of lemon and iced tea with lemon. Fruit juice is also excellent. Tea or coffee is good after lunch, but perhaps not after dinner for some. Soft drinks are generally fine, but only in *moderation—* consuming too many will significantly contribute to daily sodium.

Airline Food:
Only a Phone Call Away

A friend asked a tough question one afternoon after a discussion of low-sodium diets.

"Jim, all that's fine, but what do I eat tomorrow on the morning TWA flight to New York City?"

Stalling for time, I asked, "Are you going first class or tourist?"

Not easily bluffed, he quipped, "Wise guy!"

It's easy to call the airlines at least 24 hours before your flight and explain that you require a low-sodium meal; give them your travel time and flight number. A low-sodium meal will be given to you when the meals are served. All domestic and major foreign airlines offer this service, but you've got to give plenty of notice and follow up—the responsibility is yours.

Now that I've made it sound so easy, I've got to caution you that there are possible pitfalls in the "low-sodium" meal you're likely to get. For example, you might be served a roll or salad dressing that isn't packaged and marked "low sodium." Or a breakfast might contain sausage; that's no good. Even if you request a low-sodium meal, still apply the dos and don'ts in this chapter when there's any doubt and you'll be in fine shape.

Bring Your Own

One option that people rarely use on airlines or any commercial travel for that matter is to simply prepare their own food. The sandwiches I have described are easy to prepare; they're filling, and nutritional powerhouses. All they require is the extra effort of purchasing or making low-sodium bread, and every one is better than any airline will serve! In addition, an apple or other easily eaten fruit will give added pleasure to your trip. And you'll still be able to partake of the airline beverage service. In conclusion, it can be done if you'll only use some imagination.

Summary

You can do it! There's a wide variety of food available within our boundaries, whether you're cooking, eating out, or in the air. It's not difficult to consume less than 500 milligrams of sodium daily. Two rules apply: Eat natural foods and, when in doubt, act like a vegetarian. Nature will not let you down.

Chapter Fourteen

Basic Salt-Free Cooking

I have developed some basic recipes that help make our lives easier on a low-sodium, high–K Factor diet. There is no end to the variations that can be achieved. Some of these recipes have been adapted from standard cookbooks, some generously given by local chefs, and others adapted from an excellent book, which I highly recommend, entitled *Gourmet Cooking Without Salt* by Eleanor P. Brenner (Doubleday, 1987). Each recipe has its own character, which I have attempted to explain for your interest and enjoyment. I have emphasized sauces that make eating traditional foods more interesting and also act as vehicles for low-sodium meals (e.g., spaghetti sauce) that need livening up.

Cooking with Salt Substitutes

Recipes found in salt-free cookbooks often advocate the liberal use of salt substitutes. I am very cautiously supportive of this practice and opposed to it if the salt substitute is potassium chloride. Refresh yourself with the cautions described in Chapter Eleven. If you follow this dietary plan and use these recipes, you will get sufficient dietary potassium. If your doctor prescribes a potassium supplement to counteract your medication, you will obtain sufficient potassium from the supplement and the addition of more could be excessive. Be cautious and when in doubt go without, unless your doctor gives the okay.

If these recipes seem bland to others who are eating with you, allow them to use salt or the salt substitute. You and they also can increase zest with some of the condiments suggested here.

Zestful Flavorings

Commercial Condiments

Vegit
Lawry's Seasoned Salt-Free
Mrs. Dash
Bitters (Angostura and Underberg)
Tabasco
Poultry seasoning (salt-free)
Perc™ Seasonings (see the end of Chapter Twelve)

Herbs and Spices

Oregano
Parsley
Sage
Thyme
Chili powder (nonsalt)
Dry Mustard
Paprika
Powdered garlic

Natural Condiments

Lemon juice
Onions
Garlic, minced
Chives, minced

Basic Recipes

Recipes using many commercial and fresh foods often call for salt. These instructions must be ignored. For example, in boiling rice or cooking oatmeal, the package calls for salt. Ignore it, and to achieve the taste required seek substitutes or learn to like it salt-free. When I describe a recipe here, it is assumed that you will use no salt in cooking and a salt substitute only as required. Experiment with some of the condiments I have listed. They permit a wide variety of taste sensations, without obliterating the natural flavors of food with excess salt.

Better chefs than I have written low-sodium cookbooks, and my intention is not to even imply that I could steal their thunder. However, the recipes I have provided will familiarize you with cooking without salt and how to calculate the sodium–potassium content of foods. Also, if I could learn to prepare each of these recipes all by myself, so can you. Cooking for health can become a hobby! I urge you to purchase two books: Eleanor Brenner's *Gourmet Cooking Without Salt* and *Pennington and Church's Food Values*. Armed with these two books, you can become a great chef while making your loved ones healthy. In these recipes you will often notice that there are no sodium or potassium values given for some ingredients. This is usually done because the amount is insignificant and doesn't matter.

Low-sodium canned foods, for example, tomato sauces, mixes, and dressings, are widely available in health food stores, some gourmet shops, and large supermarkets. They are, however, expensive, and the premixed sauces, like spaghetti sauce, are often bland tasting. Therefore, I urge you, in the interest of economy and your own eating pleasure, to experiment with low-sodium cooking on your own from scratch. As long as you select ingredients that are low in sodium and natural, the potassium takes care of itself.

Once more, I caution against extensive use of salt substitutes. Some will make these and other recipes taste better, but more than about one eighth teaspoon per serving is, in my opinion, excessive and unnecessary. At that level, there should be no contraindication by your doctor.

Bread

Three kinds of breads can be made at home and used for any variety of sandwiches and meals, including toast. The three are standard white, whole wheat, and pita, or pocketbread, for sandwiches. These recipes make the equivalent of about two loaves. This convenient quantity should last long enough if two varieties are prepared at one time.

Bread making requires several basic steps that are common to all bread recipes. These can be found in just about every cookbook and, with my own variations, are summarized as follows:

1. After all the components are mixed in a large mixing bowl, a dampened dough is formed. This should be covered with a towel or plate and allowed to rest in a warm place for about 10 to 15 minutes. A warm convenient place in our house is an unused oven.
2. After resting, the dough is turned out of the bowl onto a lightly floured bread board or table (not a tiled counter), where it is kneaded for at least 10 minutes. Kneading means working it with the hands, but if you have the equipment, it can be done by

machine. Kneading should continue until the dough is smooth and elastic. Then place the dough in a large, well-buttered (not salted) bowl, being sure to roll it around so that the entire surface has been "buttered."
3. Cover the bowl with a towel, place it in a warm, draft-free place—again, an unused oven is excellent—and allow it to double in size. This step takes about 30 to 50 minutes.
4. Punch the dough down. This step is performed firmly with clenched fists by pushing the dough to the bottom of the doubling bowl. After being punched down, the dough is turned out onto a board or the table top. It can be covered with waxed paper and allowed to rest for another 10 minutes. After this, the bread is usually ready for baking. Each bread has its own baking characteristics.

White Bread

Ingredient	Sodium (mg.)	Potassium (mg.)
1 cup reconstituted low-sodium dry milk or low-sodium milk	6	617
2½ tablespoons sugar or honey	—	—
¼ cup shortening	—	—
1 cup warm water	—	—
2 packages dry yeast	8	320
2 tablespoons sugar	—	—
6 cups sifted unbleached flour	12	774
1 teaspoon white pepper	—	—
¼ cup melted unsalted butter	6	9
1 teaspoon salt substitute (optional)	—	2,800
Totals	32	4,520
Per loaf	16	2,260
Per slice	2	226
(10 slices per loaf)		
K Factor	113	

In a saucepan, scald the milk, then add the sugar (or honey) and shortening while blending with a rubber spatula or wooden spoon. Let cool to room temperature. Warm a large mixing bowl by either rinsing it in hot water and drying it or allowing it to stand in a warm (200°) oven. Pour in the warm water, yeast, 2 teaspoons sugar, and mix thoroughly until yeast has dissolved. Blend in the milk mixture with an electric blender, or by hand, then slowly blend in 3 cups of flour along with the white pepper and any salt substitute. Continue mixing, either by hand or blender, until the dough mix is smooth. Add 3 more cups of flour slowly, blending each addition completely with a wooden spoon until a smooth, damp dough is formed. Now follow the basic steps for bread preparation until the dough has been punched down and rested for 10 minutes. Divide the dough in half and place in 2 buttered 9 × 5 × 3 loaf pans. Cover the pans and put in a warm place until the dough has doubled in size, about 40 minutes to an hour. Bake the loaves in a preheated 375 degree oven for 1 hour 15 minutes or until they sound hollow when tapped with the fingers. Brush the loaves with melted butter, so they will acquire a golden brown patina when they are done. Turn the hot bread on wire racks to cool.

Whole Wheat Bread

This bread, a variation on the White Bread, substitutes whole wheat flour and molasses for white flour and sugar respectively.

Ingredient	Sodium (mg.)	Potassium (mg.)
1 cup reconstituted low-sodium dry milk or low-sodium milk	6	617
5 tablespoons blackstrap molasses	80	1,500

Ingredient	Sodium (mg.)	Potassium (mg.)
¼ cup shortening	—	—
1½ cups warm water	—	—
2 packages active dry yeast	8	20
2 tablespoons sugar	—	—
6 cups sifted whole wheat flour	24	2,664
¼ cup melted unsalted butter	6	9
1 teaspoon black pepper	—	—
1 teaspoon salt substitute (optional)	—	2,800
Totals	124	7,901
Per loaf	62	3,950
Per slice	6	395
K Factor	66	

Follow the instructions for White Bread except the first 10 minutes of baking require a higher temperature, 450 degrees, to darken the crust. Use the same techniques to determine when the bread is done.

Pita Bread

Although the Earl of Sandwich is credited with inventing the "sandwich," it really began with Middle Eastern pocket bread. This bread is such an ingenious invention I wonder why all sandwiches are not made with it. We exclusively prepare sandwiches with pita on our 47-foot ketch as we often sail on San Francisco Bay in 20 to 25 knot winds. Rough sailing and brown bagging requires a sandwich that holds together!

This pita recipe, a modification of many others, has enough flavor that it contributes to the zest of any sandwich and makes a good sandwich great.

Ingredient	Sodium (mg.)	Potassium (mg.)
2½ cups warm water	—	—
2 teaspoons sugar	—	—
2 packages active dry yeast	8	320
1½ teaspoons dry mustard	—	16
1 teaspoon white pepper	—	2
1 teaspoon salt substitute (optional)	—	—
1 tablespoon garlic powder	4	139
2 tablespoons onion powder or		
2 tablespoons dried onions	6	120
7 cups unsifted unbleached flour	14	715
Totals (15 pitas)	30	1,312
Per pita	2	87
K Factor	44	
If 1 teaspoon of salt substitute is used:		
Totals	30	4,112
Per pita	2	274
K Factor	137	

Dissolve yeast and sugar in the warm water in a large mixing bowl. Then add the mustard, pepper, salt substitute, garlic powder, and onion powder or dried onions and blend with a mixer or by hand until well mixed. Blend in slowly about 5 cups of flour until a soft smooth dough is formed. Place the remaining 1½ to 2 cups of flour on a bread board so the dough you've just made can be put on it and the remaining flour kneaded into the dough. This can be done by forming a ring with a layer of flour in the base. Knead the dough for 15 or more minutes until it is firm and clean. Follow directions for basic bread by placing dough in a covered, buttered bowl to double in size. Then punch it down and allow to double once again in the same bowl (substitute for the baking pan). When the second doubling (about 30 minutes) is complete, place it on a lightly floured bread board. Roll the dough into a slab about 5 inches wide and about 15 inches long. Divide the slab into 15 equal sections. Butter 2 or 3 baking sheets and preheat an oven to 500 degrees. Form a circle about 5 inches by ⅜ inches with each section and place on the baking sheets 3 inches apart. Bake for 10 minutes to 15 minutes until they are golden and puffed. Place on wire racks to cool.

These pitas should be large enough to form either two halves or with a segment cut off to make one large pocket. Make the pocket with a kitchen knife, slicing about ¾ through to leave a rim around the pocket. The pita dough can be formed to almost any size desired. Our experience is that the large pita is preferred. Place the pitas in a plastic bag and keep refrigerated until used.

Basic Dressings

Salads are important on this, or any other health-optimizing program. Chicken and tuna salads require mayonnaise, and green salads also need dressings. I have provided a basic plan for both. While I think these dressings are quite good, there are many others available to you either from adapting your own recipes, or borrowing from chefs who have done all the work for you. The recipes here should get you started, however.

Mayonnaise

Mayonnaise is essential for chicken, shrimp, tuna, and other salads, and sandwiches in general. It simply consists of eggs, oil, and seasonings. There is a critical step: adding oil to the mix while it is being blended. This recipe is my composite of several recipes and makes a little over a cup of "plain" mayonnaise that keeps for two weeks. *Gourmet Cooking Without Salt* provides excellent mayonnaise recipes with varied flavors that enhance many other foods calling for mayonnaise.

Ingredient	Sodium (mg.)	Potassium (mg.)
1 large egg plus a yolk	69	65
1 tablespoon fresh lemon juice	—	19
¼ teaspoon dry mustard	—	11
¼ teaspoon salt substitute (optional)	—	1,540
½ teaspoon sugar	—	—
⅛ teaspoon cayenne pepper	1	5
⅛ teaspoon white pepper	—	—
Mix ½ cup olive oil and ½ cup corn oil together		
Totals (makes 1 cup)	70	1,635
Per tablespoon	4	102
K Factor	25	

Hold back the oil and blend all the other ingredients at low speed. Then, at low speed, add the oil slowly through the top of the blender so that the oil is blended as it is introduced. This step takes about 30 seconds and produces a thick, creamy mayonnaise. Note that the oil must be added slowly and be blended completely or the oil will separate from the mayonnaise. I suggest you try this mayonnaise without a salt substitute and use a dash each of garlic powder and onion powder.

Soybean Mayonnaise

This mayonnaise, in contrast to the one made from eggs, is completely cholesterol free, lower in sodium, and very low in fat. It is excellent on any dietary program to improve health.

Ingredient	Sodium (mg.)	Potassium (mg.)
6 ounces tofu (soybean curd), pressed between towels to remove liquid	14	84
2 tablespoons lemon juice	1	38
2 tablespoons olive oil, mixed with	—	—
1 tablespoon corn oil		
¼ teaspoon dry mustard	—	—
Totals	15	122
K Factor	8	

In blender, combine tofu, juice, and mustard; then, with blender at low speed, add olive oil and corn oil mixture slowly to make a creamy consistency. Store tightly in refrigerator; it tastes best in about four days, but can be used immediately.

Basic Salad Dressing

Salads are essential to this dietary plan and for good health in general, and salad dressing makes the salad. This basic dressing will keep indefinitely when refrigerated, and can be taken with you on an airline flight, for example, when you know you'll need a salad dressing.

Ingredient	Sodium (mg.)	Potassium (mg.)
1 cup olive oil (for gourmet use, substitute walnut or avocado oil)	—	—
¼ cup cider vinegar (wine vinegar or other vinegars are acceptable)	—	—
1 teaspoon black pepper	—	—
3 cloves pressed garlic	—	—
Dash of onion powder	—	—
	Sodium–Potassium is negligible	

Blend all ingredients in a bowl with a wire whisk. After preparation, this dressing should be stored in a covered jar so it can be shaken before using.

Breakfast Foods

Breakfast starts the day right. I have provided two cereal müsli recipes that should satisfy any gourmet. But pancakes, waffles, and omelets offer a greater challenge. Seek recipes and low-sodium mixes for these foods.

Granola Cereal

This granola is an excellent snack all by itself, makes a great cereal with milk, and müsli when blended with plain yogurt.

Ingredient	Sodium (mg.)	Potassium (mg.)
¼ cup raisins	18	1,119
3 dates, chopped	1	162
½ cup water	—	—
2 large, very ripe bananas	10	554
1 tablespoon vanilla	—	—
8 cups rolled oats	1	1,056
½ cup raw, unsalted sunflower seeds	32	1,032
1 cup chopped walnuts, hazelnuts, pinenuts, or unsalted almonds	16	536
2 teaspoons cinnamon	—	—
Totals	78	4,459
Per serving	8	445
K Factor	56	

Soak raisins and dates in water until plump. Mash bananas with raisins and dates. Stir in vanilla. Mix dry ingredients. Add the banana mixture to the mixed dry ingredients. Spread on cookie sheets and bake at 200 degrees until light brown and dry. Store dry in cannister. Makes 10 servings of cereal.

Scala's Oatmeal Müsli

A breakfast of grains and fruit without milk follows in the European tradition of müsli. My use of it evolved from a previous book for people with arthritis who had to avoid milk. It tastes excellent, is healthy, and allows almost endless variation in preparation. The following recipe makes two servings.

Ingredient	Sodium (mg.)	Potassium (mg.)
⅔ cup rolled oats	—	88
1 cup cold water	—	—
½ cup apricot nectar	5	143
⅓ cup raisins (optional)	6	375
Additional apricot nectar if desired		
Totals	11	606
K Factor	55	

Add oats to the cold water and apricot nectar along with the raisins. Cook over low heat, stirring frequently until mixture comes to a boil. Cover; remove from heat. Let stand until desired consistency. To serve, simply add additional apricot nectar for liquid. The müsli should require no further sweetening. Fresh or dried fruits and nuts can be added as desired.

Puff Pancakes

Pancakes are a major problem on a low-sodium diet because they require both baking soda and baking powder.

It is possible to get salt-free baking powder, but I haven't been able to find salt-free baking soda. If you can obtain both, you can substitute them in standard recipes. I have modified a recipe that permits a wide latitude for the pancake lover, however.

Ingredient	Sodium (mg.)	Potassium (mg.)
4 egg yolks	32	60
¼ cup cold water	—	—
¼ cup unsifted flour	1	32
¼ teaspoon salt substitute	—	700
4 egg whites	200	180
Totals	233	972
K Factor	4	

Beat the egg yolks until thick. Add the water, flour, salt substitute, and beat until smooth. Beat egg whites until stiff. Fold in the stiffly beaten egg whites until the entire batter is smooth.

Drop the batter by spoonsful on a hot, well-greased griddle; turn when lightly brown. Serve with syrup or fruit syrup made by blending frozen fruit (strawberries, blueberries, or peaches) into maple syrup.

Variations of these pancakes use cooked rice, wheat germ, or minced potatoes. Add ½ cup of one of these ingredients, fold into the mix with the stiffened egg whites, and prepare in the same way. Another variation adds apple slices, blueberries, or strawberry halves to the pancake just after it has been dropped on the grill.

Soup

People used to describe an unsuccessful person by saying, "He can't afford salt for soup." Now, I consider a person

who can make a good soup without salt or salt substitute
successful. It's not easy. A simple technique is to add
Tabasco, ginger, and other spices to low-sodium soups.
Two "basic" soups are provided here. Once you can serve
low-sodium soup to your friends and get compliments, you
have become a successful low-sodium chef.

Creamy Tomato Soup

This modification of a recipe from the Domaine Chandon
Winery of Napa Valley is normally served in a pastry shell.
You can serve it in a bowl, garnished with chopped chives,
parsley, or grated carrots, and enjoy many compliments.
This recipe provides six servings.

Ingredient	Sodium (mg.)	Potassium (mg.)
2 16-ounce cans of salt-free tomatoes or 2 pounds of ripe tomatoes, chopped coarsely	28	2,215
1 medium onion, chopped	10	157
1 tablespoon butter	2	3
1 tablespoon brown sugar or honey	—	—
2 teaspoons finely chopped basil	1	96
½ teaspoon salt substitute	1	192
Dash (four drops) Tabasco sauce	—	—
½ teaspoon pepper	2	2
1 pint half and half	192	512
1 cup double-strength reconstituted low-sodium dry milk	16	1,232
2 tablespoons chopped chives	2	50
½ teaspoon grated ginger	1	12
Totals	255	4,471
Per serving	42	745
K Factor	17	

Peel and seed the tomatoes. Sauté the onion in the butter over medium heat (do not brown). Add chopped tomatoes, sugar, basil, salt substitute, Tabasco sauce, pepper, and ginger. Simmer for about 25 minutes. Use mixer or blender to puree the simmered contents. Strain. Add half and half and reconstituted milk. Garnish with chopped chives, parsley, or grated carrots.

Gazpacho

Ingredient	Sodium (mg.)	Potassium (mg.)
3 large tomatoes, peeled and chopped	18	1,464
1 green pepper, chopped	13	213
1 cucumber, peeled and chopped	6	160
1 cup celery, chopped	126	341
½ cup onion, chopped	7	116
4 cups no-sodium tomato juice	6	598
If not available, make tomato juice by juicing tomatoes and straining through a colander.		
2 avocados, chopped	42	2,194
¼ cup red wine vinegar	—	—
¼ cup olive oil	—	—
½ teaspoons salt substitute	1	192
½ teaspoon black pepper	1	13
½ teaspoon grated ginger	1	12
6 cloves garlic, very finely chopped	6	186
8 drops Tabasco sauce	—	—
Totals	227	5,489
Per serving	28	686
K Factor	24	

All the vegetables must be finely chopped and the ingredients placed in the bowl for 12 hours before serving. It is important that this soup be prepared in a nonmetallic bowl;

plastic or china bowls are essential. Served cold, it makes an excellent summer appetizer.
Yield: 8 servings.

Sauces for Pasta

I have developed sauces for the pleasure of eating pasta, rice, and seafood. These sauces are basic and permit much flexibility. With a little imagination and experimentation, they can greatly enhance your eating horizons.

Basic Tomato Sauce

Pasta makes an excellent meal for this program, but pasta is only as good as its sauce. Good tomato sauce can be prepared without salt. Starting with salt-free canned plum tomatoes is best, but they are not always available, nor are fresh plum tomatoes, so I have provided several options for them. Always remember that a spaghetti sauce permits wide variation in preparation, so be flexible and inventive with ingredients; use spices and herbs to suit your taste.

Ingredient	Sodium (mg.)	Potassium (mg.)
3 tablespoons olive oil	—	—
1 medium onion, chopped	10	157
4 garlic cloves, chopped	1	16
2 16-ounce cans salt-free plum tomatoes or 24 fresh plum or Romano tomatoes, or about 6 medium sized tomatoes	28	2,215
1 can salt-free tomato paste	100	2,237
1 can salt-free tomato sauce	20	389
1 cup water	—	—
⅛ teaspoon cayenne	—	—
3 teaspoons sugar	—	—

Ingredient	Sodium (mg.)	Potassium (mg.)
1 bay leaf	—	—
2 tablespoons parsley, finely chopped	8	146
1 large carrot, grated	47	341
½ teaspoon pepper	1	13
1 teaspoon basil	1	48
½ teaspoon oregano	—	12
Totals	188	5,574
Per serving	31	929
K Factor	30	

Chop tomatoes briefly in a blender. Combine ingredients in a large pot. Simmer covered for 1 to 2 hours. Add salt substitute only if absolutely necessary. More or less garlic and onion can be used depending upon the taste of the people being served.
Yield: About 6 servings

Preparing Pasta

Pasta should be placed in a large volume of boiling water to which at least one tablespoon of olive oil has been added. Do not add salt as package directions state. Boil, with occasional stirring, to the desired level of tenderness, strain, and serve.

Ingredient	Sodium (mg.)	Potassium (mg.)
Pasta, 1 cup	1	115
Sauce	31	929
Totals	32	1,044
K Factor	33	

Basic Clam Sauce

Another excuse for pasta—clam sauce! When made without cream, it is a terrific vehicle for pasta and provides an excellent protein, high-carbohydrate, low-fat meal. Clam sauce is best when served with a salad and a light Frascati wine. This sauce is modified from my grandmother's basic recipe.

A problem that must be overcome from this sauce is the chopped clams. Chopped clams canned with salt cannot be used. If you can get them without salt, there's no problem. There are two other means available: Steam either refrigerated or frozen clams. This recipe requires about 6 medium or 4 large clams per serving, about 24 clams total.

If you are *not* using canned clams, steam the clams on a steamer rack for 8 to 10 minutes in a large pot with 1 cup water. Use seasonings such as bay leaves, oregano, parsley, shaved carrots, and a glass of white wine. When they're done, most of the clams will open; save the broth.

Remove the clams from the shell; chop on a cutting board into bite-sized or smaller pieces. Set aside for the sauce.

Ingredient	Sodium (mg.)	Potassium (mg.)
3 tablespoons olive oil	—	—
1 medium onion, minced	10	157
2 cloves garlic, minced	—	—
8 to 10 ounces clam broth	—	—
½ cup dry white wine	7	84
1 tablespoon parsley, minced	4	73
¼ teaspoon white pepper	—	—
2 tablespoons unsalted butter	—	—
24 clams, minced	216	1,416
Totals	237	1,730
Per serving	59	432
K Factor	7	
K Factor (with pasta)	9	

Heat oil in a skillet. Add onion and garlic, and sauté over medium heat until golden. Add clam broth, stir in wine, simmer over medium heat. While simmering, add chopped clams, parsley, pepper, and butter; continue simmering for 5 to 10 minutes.

Pour sauce over hot cooked linguini, vermicelli, fettucine, or spaghetti. Mix thoroughly with wooden serving spoons, and serve. If fresh clams are used, one or two can be used as a nice garnish atop each dish. Traditional clam sauce has the clams mixed in the pasta, however. You can put a little parsley on top to dress it up.

Red Clam Sauce

Use the basic tomato sauce and add the steamed minced clams. Allow the sauce to simmer uncovered for about an hour and you have a great red clam sauce.

Six Main Dishes

I have included five dishes that make excellent low-sodium, high–K Factor meals of traditional foods. They teach that special dietary foods can be as appetizing as any gourmet foods. Indeed, two have been adapted from recipes given to me by two of California's finest restaurants; they are served every day with compliments to the chef.

Chicken with Broccoli and Cashews

This spectacular dish is a modification of one of our favorite "wok" dishes. It normally requires soy sauce, but I developed a modification with Angostura bitters that retains the same flavor without sodium.

Ingredient	Sodium (mg.)	Potassium (mg.)
1 tablespoon cornstarch	—	—
1 cup low-sodium chicken broth (can also be made from two low-sodium chicken bouillon cubes)	5	—
⅓ cup dry sherry	2	45
2 dashes Angostura bitters	—	—
½ teaspoon Tabasco sauce	11	2
¼ cup olive oil	—	—
3 chicken breasts, skinned, boned, and cut into 1-inch pieces	408	1,422
½ teaspoon grated ginger	1	—
3 cups broccoli flowerets	126	1,344
1 large red sweet pepper cut into 1-inch squares	13	213
½ pound mushrooms, sliced	34	939
1 bunch green onions, slivered	5	231
3 cloves garlic, minced	—	—
⅓ cup dry roasted cashews, unsalted	2	70
Totals	607	4,266
Per serving	101	711
K Factor	7	

Combine cornstarch, chicken broth, sherry, bitters, and Tabasco sauce in a small bowl and set aside. Ten minutes before serving, heat olive oil in large skillet or wok. When oil is very hot, add chicken and ginger. Cook about 3 minutes, stirring and turning constantly until chicken is white. Remove chicken to a bowl on side. In some woks it can be placed on a rack.

Place the broccoli, red pepper, mushrooms, onions, and garlic in same wok and cook for 3 to 5 minutes, stirring constantly. Add back the chicken, then pour in the cornstarch mixture, and stir constantly until the sauce thickens. Add in the cashews.

Serve over steaming hot white or brown rice. This dish is especially good over steaming hot wild rice.
Yield: 6 servings

Scampi-Style Prawns Italiano

This recipe from Flaherty's Restaurant in Carmel, California, was a low-sodium recipe that I could use with one minor modification. It is most appropriately served on a bed of linguini.

Ingredient	Sodium (mg.)	Potassium (mg.)
Salt-free butter for sautéing	—	—
Flour for dredging, seasoned with pepper	—	—
24 large prawns, about ½ pound, peeled and deveined	318	500
1 tablespoon fresh garlic, finely chopped	1	9
1 tablespoon fresh chopped shallots	6	167
½ cup dry white wine	7	84
12 quartered artichoke hearts	80	420
⅔ cup tomatoes, diced	3	382
3 tablespoons capers, drained	—	—
1 cup fresh mushrooms, sliced	15	414
½ cup green onions, diced	4	70
½ teaspoon ginger, grated	1	12
Totals	435	2,054
Per serving	109	513
K Factor	5	

Dredge prawns in the seasoned flour. Heat butter over high heat, add prawns, and sauté, turning frequently, for two minutes. Immediately add garlic and shallots. Add wine and ignite either with a match or by tilting pan toward burner. When flame is extinguished, add remaining ingredients. Reduce heat and simmer for two minutes more.

Prepare 20 ounces of linguine or fettucine (no salt in cooking) and divide into four portions. Divide the sauce and prawns evenly over the pasta. Garnish each plate with chopped parsley.

Yield: 4 servings

Hogback Pork Chops

This dish, with fat trimmed, is not excessive in fat and makes an excellent, festive, low-sodium, high–K Factor meal. Its ingredients and preparation make it a favorite with children; the entire family can enjoy a very healthy meal.

Ingredient	Sodium (mg.)	Potassium (mg.)
8 pork chops	480	4,544
½ cup apple juice	4	143
⅔ cup plumped raisins	12	751
6 drops Tabasco sauce	15	—
¼ cup brown sugar	17	161
¼ teaspoon nutmeg	—	4
¼ teaspoon cinnamon	—	4
4 large apples, each cut into 6 or 8 wedges (Pippin are best and Yellow Delicious are good)	4	636
½ cup water	—	—
Totals	532	6,243
Per serving	66	780
K Factor	12	

Brown the chops in a skillet over medium heat and remove. Arrange browned chops in a shallow 2-quart baking dish and pour in apple juice, Tabasco sauce, and raisins. Cover and bake at 350 degrees for 45 minutes.

While chops are baking, coat apples with the brown sugar, nutmeg, and cinnamon mixture, making more if necessary. Turn chops in baking dish, arrange apple wedges around the chops, and sprinkle the entire dish with the brown sugar, nutmeg, cinnamon mixture. Pour ½ cup water over entire contents. Cover and bake for 15 minutes.

This dish is best served with wild rice, but white rice is also excellent.

Yield: 8 servings.

Avocado Tuna Salad

Avocados are an unsung fruit that, when ripe, substitute for mayonnaise in our house and on our boat. This particular salad is equally good with chicken chunks, turkey white meat, or crabmeat.

Ingredient	Sodium (mg.)	Potassium (mg.)
6½ ounces low-sodium chunk tuna	72	478
1 avocado, very ripe	21	1,097
½ tomato	2	183
½ medium onion, chopped	5	77
1 teaspoon lemon juice (more if desired)	0	6
1 tablespoon parsley, chopped	4	73
¾ tablespoon cider vinegar	—	—
Totals	104	1,914
Per serving	26	478
K Factor	18	

Combine the ingredients in a bowl and blend thoroughly with a large fork. Taste can be altered by adding, as preferred, Tabasco sauce, horseradish, or chopped chili peppers. This salad is excellent when served as a sandwich in low-sodium pita bread.
Yield: 4 servings

Kettle of Fish

A dish that works with any fish fillet and is completely foolproof. It is best with flounder, haddock, or sole, but also works well with sea bass and red snapper. It is excellent with frozen fish fillets.

Ingredient	Sodium (mg.)	Potassium (mg.)
3 large potatoes peeled and thinly sliced	18	2,265
½ pound fresh mushrooms, sliced	34	939
1 pound zucchini in ⅛ inch slices	8	828
4 large tomatoes, peeled, seeded, and sliced	24	1,952
4 green onions, thinly sliced	40	628
1½ pounds fish fillets	370	2,488
2 tablespoons salt-free butter, melted	—	—
½ teaspoon thyme	1	7
½ teaspoon basil	—	24
½ teaspoon oregano	—	12
½ teaspoon ground ginger in two ¼ teaspoon divisions	1	12
½ teaspoon black pepper	1	13
1 tablespoon parsley, chopped	4	73
½ lemon, sliced	1	40
Totals	502	9,281
Per serving	84	1,546
K Factor	18	

Generously butter an oblong baking dish. Arrange sliced potatoes on bottom and sprinkle with ¼ teaspoon ground ginger. Cover with foil and bake at 350 degrees for 15 minutes. Place other vegetables over the partially cooked potatoes and layer the fish fillets on top. Cut a few diagonal slashes in the fillets.

Sprinkle the remaining herbs and the remaining ginger on the fish. Sprinkle the black pepper evenly over the fish. Return to oven and bake 20 more minutes or until fish is either browned or flakes easily. Garnish with lemon slices and parsley and serve.

Yield: 4 to 6 servings

Bahamian Fillet

This dish appears under many titles. It originated in the British West Indies, where it originally called for molasses. This low-sodium modification is virtually indistinguishable from the original. Traditionally sole fillet is used. The recipe works well, however, with haddock and red or gray snapper.

Ingredient	Sodium (mg.)	Potassium (mg.)
1½ pounds fillet of sole (4 fillets)	383	2,511
¼ cup flour	—	—
¼ teaspoon white pepper	—	—
1 teaspoon paprika	—	—
½ teaspoon ginger	—	—
5 tablespoons unsalted butter	—	—
½ cup dry white wine	7	84
2 tablespoons lemon juice	—	38
2 tablespoons molasses, or brown sugar	32	600
2 large bananas cut in quarters lengthwise	2	902
Totals	425	4,168
Per serving	106	1,042
K Factor	10	

Dredge the fillets in the flour, paprika, and white pepper. Melt butter in large skillet and brown the fillets for about 3 minutes on each side over medium heat. Remove to a warm platter.

Combine wine, ginger, lemon juice, and molasses in skillet. Add bananas and cook over a medium-high heat for about 2 minutes while spooning the sauce over the bananas. Cover the fillets with the bananas and the sauce. Garnish with parsley or slivered almonds.

This dish is delicious with wild rice and does very well with steaming white rice. A green salad or other fresh green vegetable is appropriate.

Yield: 4 servings

Side Dishes

Fruit Powerhouse

This is undoubtedly the simplest of all cranberry recipes. It is very flexible, goes well as a relish with just about any poultry dish, and makes an excellent salad if served on a bed of lettuce. It also goes very well with vanilla ice cream.

Ingredient	Sodium (mg.)	Potassium (mg.)
1 pound bag fresh cranberries	5	335
2 seedless oranges with the skin	2	500
1 large apple, cored	1	159
2 cups crushed pineapple with juice	2	350
Honey to taste	—	—
Totals	10	1,344
Per serving	1	134
K Factor	134	

In the blender, blend all the ingredients and add honey to desired sweetness. Alternatives to honey are maple syrup or sugar. If you use sugar, some water might be necessary. The final result should be spoonable and hold its shape. Yield: About 10 servings

Carrot Cabbage Powerhouse

This dish, from my mother, is often served as a dessert in our house, topped with sour cream, yogurt, or whipped cream. It's easy to make and doesn't taste like special-diet food.

Ingredient	Sodium (mg.)	Potassium (mg.)
1 package lemon-flavored Jell-O, 6-ounce size	—	—
2 cups boiling water	—	—
1 cup cold water	—	—
1 cup lemon juice	1	150
¼ head shredded green cabbage	40	466
¼ head shredded red cabbage	26	268
2 large carrots shredded	94	682
Totals	161	1,566
Per serving	16	156
K Factor	10	

Dissolve Jell-O in boiling water; then add cold water and lemon juice. Refrigerate until slightly jelled. Stir in shredded cabbage and carrots and refrigerate until firmly set. Yield: 10 servings

Desserts

Two things are necessary for good low-sodium, high–K Factor desserts: piecrusts and cake recipes. Once a piecrust is made, your options are unlimited. I strongly urge you to use a good picture cookbook if you are inexperienced. I favor *Betty Crocker*, but *Better Homes and Gardens* is equally good.

Piecrust

This pie shell is an adaptation of several crusts. I can't emphasize enough the value of Eleanor Brenner's *Gourmet Cooking Without Salt*, which contains such detailed instructions that anyone can produce a low-sodium pie crust every time.

Ingredient	Sodium (mg.)	Potassium (mg.)
For each pie shell:		
½ cup all-purpose flour	1	65
½ cup whole wheat flour	1	52
¼ cup unsalted butter, cut in small pieces	—	—
¼ teaspoon salt substitute	—	700
3 tablespoons cold water	—	—
Totals	2	817
K Factor		408

Sift flour and salt substitute together. Cut in small pieces of butter with sharp knives or with a pastry blender. Add 2 tablespoons water and stir with a fork until the dough begins to stick together. Add more cold water sparingly if needed to get dough into a uniform ball. Let ball rest at least 10 minutes and it can be refrigerated overnight.

Roll dough out between two sheets of wax paper. Remove one waxed paper and fit dough into a glass pie dish. Then remove the second wax paper carefully.

Partially bake at 400 degrees for 7 minutes; for a chiffon pie, bake completely at 400 degrees for 12 minutes; for fruit pie, bake with the pie.

Apple Pie

This apple pie is an example of the pies that can be made and used on this program. Apple pie calls for a top crust that can be made in the same way as the bottom crust. Simply remove one waxed paper and place over the filling; then, very gently, remove the top paper.

Ingredient	Sodium (mg.)	Potassium (mg.)
7 large or 9 medium tart apples, cut into slices (Pippin or Yellow Delicious)	9	1,431
2 tablespoons fresh lemon juice	6	30
½ cup brown sugar	34	322
1½ tablespoons cornstarch	—	—
2 teaspoons cinnamon	2	22
½ teaspoon ground nutmeg	—	8
2 tablespoons unsalted butter, shaved into small slivers	—	—
2 piecrusts are required		
Total, filling only	51	1,813
Total, crusts	4	1,634
Totals	55	3,447
Serving (⅛ of pie)	7	430
K Factor	61	

Place apples in a bowl; add lemon juice and sugar, and toss the apples to mix. Then add cornstarch, nutmeg, and cinnamon with continued mixing so everything is well blended. Layer the apples into a piecrust in a Pyrex pie dish. Put the butter shavings on the apples liberally and equally. Cover the dish with the top crust. Trim and flute the crust along the edges. Prick the top crust with a fork in 5 or 6 places. Bake the pie for 10 minutes at 450 degrees; then reduce the heat to 350 degrees and bake for 50 minutes until the crust is golden brown.

Lemon Chiffon Pie

This is a favorite, modest in calories, low in sodium, and very easy to prepare. It lends itself to the addition of strawberries or other fruit. Adding fruit not only increases variety, it also increases the potassium content.

This same recipe can be used to make orange, lime, and pineapple chiffon pies. Simply substitute the other fruit for lemons. Fruit pieces can be folded in when the components are combined, for example, strawberries or kiwi wedges.

Ingredient	Sodium (mg.)	Potassium (mg.)
Baked pie shell	2	817
½ cup sugar	—	—
1 envelope unflavored gelatin	8	180
⅔ cup water	—	—
⅓ cup lemon juice	1	101
4 egg yolks, slightly beaten	32	60
1 tablespoon grated lemon rind	—	10
Totals	43	1,168
Serving (⅛ of pie)	5	146
K Factor	29	

Thoroughly blend everything except the lemon rind in a saucepan. Over a medium heat stir constantly until it starts to boil. Just as it starts to boil, blend in the grated lemon

rind and place saucepan in a pan of cold water until the mixture mounds when dropped from a spoon.
Now prepare meringue:

4 egg whites
½ cup sugar
½ teaspoon cream of tartar

Beat egg whites with cream of tartar until frothy. Slowly beat in sugar until it is blended well and the meringue is stiff and glossy.
Combine the filling with the meringue. Fold the filling from the saucepan into the meringue and gently mix until thoroughly blended. Pour into a baked pie shell and refrigerate for several hours until thoroughly set.

Carrot Cake

Carrot cake is traditional, healthy, and flexible. You can add raisins, prune pieces, nuts, and even chopped dates to a carrot cake and it turns out all right. This cake is moist.

Ingredient	Sodium (mg.)	Potassium (mg.)
2½ cups grated carrots	190	808
1 cup unbleached flour	2	129
6 teaspoons salt-free baking powder	—	—
1 teaspoon cinnamon	—	—
1 teaspoon allspice	—	—
2 eggs	138	130
¾ cup corn oil	—	—
1 cup sugar	—	—
1 cup raisins	18	1,126
1 cup chopped pecans (80 halves)	8	419
Totals	356	2,612
Serving (⅛ of cake)	45	326
K Factor	7	

Sift flour, baking powder, cinnamon, and nutmeg. Beat eggs with corn oil until thoroughly blended. Add sugar while continuing to beat until mixed.

Slowly beat in the flour, cinnamon, nutmeg mixture until it is thoroughly blended. With a spatula, fold in the carrots, raisins, and chopped pecans and mix thoroughly.

Bake in a loaf pan or a round bundt pan. I prefer a 9 × 5 glass dish. The pan should be thoroughly buttered. Bake at 350 degrees for 40 to 50 minutes.

Strawberry Mousse

Mousse desserts go well at any dinner and with any group. This mousse is made in two parts; the mousse and the sauce.

Mousse Ingredient	Sodium (mg.)	Potassium (mg.)
4 cups strawberries	8	988
1 cup sugar (brown is okay)	—	—
¼ cup water with ¼ teaspoon cream of tartar	—	—
6 egg yolks	48	90
¼ cup Grand Marnier	—	—
1 cup whipping cream	—	—
Sauce		
1 cup strawberries	2	247
1 cup raspberries or another cup of strawberries will do	0	180
½ cup sugar	—	—
1 cup sliced strawberries	2	247
3 tablespoons Grand Marnier	—	—
Totals	60	1,752
Serving	7	219
K Factor	29	

Mousse Preparation
Puree strawberries and set aside.

In a saucepan, combine water with cream of tartar, add sugar, and bring to a boil and cook until sugar is dissolved. Add strawberry puree and continue to cook for about 5 minutes.

In a large mixing bowl, beat the egg yolks until smooth, pour in the strawberry syrup from preceding step, and beat the mixture until it is cool. Add the Grand Marnier.

Whip the cream until it holds peaks and fold into the strawberry blend. Chill this bowl of mousse.

Sauce Preparation
Puree strawberries and raspberries in a blender with sugar for 30 seconds. Transfer the puree to a saucepan, add strawberry slices, bring to a boil, remove strawberry slices with a slotted spoon, and simmer sauce until thickened. Put strawberry slices in a bowl and pour the thickened sauce over them. Add the Grand Marnier.

Cover the sauce and allow to chill.

Assembly
Spoon a layer of sauce into 8 parfait glasses. Fill the glasses ⅓ full with mousse; add more sauce, then more mousse. Top with whipped cream.

Additional Reading

Choices for a Healthy Heart
Piscatella, Joseph C.
Workman, 1987

Gourmet Cooking Without Salt
Brenner, Eleanor P.
Doubleday, 1987

Light Style, The New American Cuisine
Dosti, Rose; Kidushim, Deborah; Wolke, Mark
Harper & Row, 1982

Salt-Free Cooking with Herbs and Spices
Roth, June
Contemporary Books, 1975

The Control Your High Blood Pressure Cookbook
Bennett, Cleaves M., M.D., and Newport, Cristine
Doubleday, 1987

Section Three

Lifestyle

Prologue

The Texture of Life

Lifestyle becomes the texture of your life. It's what you choose to be. I'm going to ask you to create a texture that makes a statement. The statement is, "This body is me and I want it to be as sound and healthy as it can be." I like to think of it in one word—optimize.

Three statements that characterize this concept are:

What you visualize for yourself you become.
What you think, you are.
What you think, you do.

I always think of a friend I know, Bob Sissler, who lost his sight while in the Air Force. He went on to get his Ph.D., took to skiing, became an excellent fly fisherman, and above all enjoyed a healthy life. He did his very best with his body and optimized everything about himself, especially his health. Think of this blind man downhill skiing if you ever get the urge to say, "I can't do it."

In this section you'll assess your weight and make a commitment to either losing or staying the same. If you want to lose, I'll explore a simple plan that works, and you won't have to diet.

251

You will evaluate your internal and external stress. External stress can come from many sources, from the household pet to a boss who wants you out. Internal stress is what the name implies; you'll have to assess yourself. Whether you're under internal or external stress, we'll explore the concepts of positive thinking. We'll identify the need to greet your fellow man with a smile, to have the serenity to know you're doing your best, giving and receiving love.

Recent research has proven that the old saying, "It's in your head," is to some extent correct. Studies have indicated that some people can, with a little mental effort, cause their blood pressure to drop. This, combined with diet and a little exercise, should add up to total control.

Exercise helps the body to cope with any stress, but it's absolutely essential to help reduce high blood pressure. Don't worry if you're not an athlete; exercise shouldn't be hard, just significant enough and consistent to do some good. Exercise benefits every aspect of your health. Indeed, recent research has shown that it even reduces the risk for cancer. But the most important outcome is its positive effect on mental outlook. It's got everything in its favor and nothing against it.

Chapter Fifteen

Fit or Fat

Many hypertensives can cure themselves by simply pushing away from the table a little sooner at each meal. In Chapter Five, I explained that overweight, in some people, places an insulin stress on the kidney and indirectly causes high blood pressure. Also, I pointed out that some high blood pressure is simply the increased amount of force the heart must produce to push blood through all that flab. In defiance of all our understanding, however, there are grossly overweight people with normal blood pressure. How do normal folks weave their way through this maze to know what to do?

Overweight has nothing in its favor. In fact, overweight people have a shorter life expectancy and get more diseases than average. Most important, they are at greater risk for heart disease, cancer, and stroke. If the overweight is complicated by high blood pressure and bad habits like drinking or smoking, the risk of an early death gets much greater. And the quality of life declines even more.

Now, I'm sure you know of someone who was always big as a house, smoked, drank, watched television incessantly, and lived to be 92, but I can assure you that if your acquaintance hadn't done all that, he or she would probably have lived to be 102 or more. Being overweight simply doesn't have anything in its favor, and has many things against it. Most important for our purposes is that a person with high blood pressure should not be overweight.

How Much to Weigh

Overweight is an overworked term! It implies that there is some arbitrary standard that tells precisely how much you should weigh. An "ideal" weight can be established by setting a level for your body fat in concert with your life-style. This is what I call the "Certified Public Accounting" of weight determination. It requires that you have yourself weighed under water and on land. Since fat floats, the difference is how much your fat weighs; and the weight of your fat, divided by your land weight, gives your percentage of body fat.

If you're an average man, in good shape, you'll have 13% to 15% body fat; you likely get some active exercise, some tennis or jogging, for example, and would be able to run a mile in under 8.5 minutes.

If you're an average woman in good shape, you'll have 20% to 22% body fat. Like your average male colleague, you probably get moderate exercise and can run a mile (or equivalent) in under 8.5 minutes without difficulty.

By comparison, if you were a regular distance runner, I would expect you to come in at 8% or 9% body fat and wouldn't be surprised at 6% for serious marathoners. If you were a fast-moving tennis player, about 13% would be normal for men, about 15% for women. I think you get the idea from this that percentage of body fat is proportionate to physical need up to a point, and fat beyond that percentage is just too much fat. And too much fat imposes stress on your heart, other organs, joints, and in many people causes high blood pressure.

The difference between dry land weight and wet weight also gives you your lean body mass. That's the weight of everything else: your bones, muscles, teeth, tendons—everything. Lean body mass requires more metabolic energy than fat. You can see this difference for yourself by inspecting a steak before it's trimmed, with fat still on its periphery. The red meat (muscle) contains blood vessels and much fiber, while the fat is lacking in blood vessels and is as uniform as a stick of butter. Obviously, the muscle is very active tissue and fat is very passive. Also, throw it into water—this cut floats, lean meat doesn't.

At the other end, albeit rare, is the specter of under-weight. Serious underweight is a medical problem often more dangerous than obesity. People who are seriously underweight have shorter life expectancies, just as over-weight people do. So, the concept of maintaining a reason-able weight for your body makes sense from either direction.

Body Changes As We Age

When we're young, our lean body mass is considerable. We are more active, and the energy necessary to maintain everything is higher. As we age, our need for muscle mass usually declines and the energy necessary to keep every-thing working declines in proportion. The energy we need to keep functioning is called the basal metabolism, and it declines normally with age. If everything remained propor-tional, our weight would decline as well, because our fat content would be maintained at a constant percentage, say 22% for a woman.

Unfortunately, our lifestyle goes against us. Eating habits are usually established in the teenage years and activity levels drop off as we enter the work force after school. Therefore, energy expenditure as exercise and work de-clines, while we consume the same food calories. We usu-ally consume more calories as we get older; for example, meals and snacks become longer, more regular, and are likely to be enhanced with alcohol. Consequently, people usually gain weight as they get older, and it's very, very rare that their body fat percentage declines. Indeed, per-centage of body fat usually increases as people get older.

For example, thirteen years after marriage the average woman has gained 23 pounds and the average man 18 pounds. If you accept 25 as the average marriage age, thirteen years later, age 38, is when high blood pressure seems to get started.

I can summarize this for you by pointing out that as we get older, our weight should slowly decline unless we are very active. For example, if you're a man and lean body mass was 140 pounds at 20 when very active, you simply don't require that same lean body mass at age 50 even if you jog 10 miles weekly. Nor should your percentage of body fat be any different. Let me illustrate with an example.

	Man—15% Fat		
Age	**Lean Body Mass**	**% Fat**	**Total Weight**
20	140	15	165
40	135	15	158
60	130	15	153

Unfortunately, in our society, the man in my illustration at age 20 is much more likely to be over 175, and possibly as high as 190 at age 40 and more at 60. All this tells us that lifestyle changes, accompanied by human biology, cause weight to increase, not decrease, as we get older. So, how do you deal with your weight if you've got high blood pressure? First, let's decide whether or not you're overweight.

A Personal Weight Assessment

If it's possible for you to have your percentage of body fat precisely determined, by all means have it done, because you can determine very accurately how much weight, if any, you should lose. There are two methods commonly used and I'll give you a third.

The first method, weighing both in and out of water, is the most direct and most precise. It requires sophisticated equipment, however, and can't be done at home, or even in the doctor's office unless he's a sophisticated weight-loss specialist. Actually, you can weigh yourself quite accurately in the water if you are willing to get a spring-type bathroom scale wet and have the use of a pool. All you've got to do is weigh yourself (in bathing suit) on the ground; then take the scale into the pool and do the same thing with as little of you out of the water as possible and after breathing out. It can be done if you'll simply duck your head under to read the numbers on the scale and hold as little breath as possible. It's a lot of trouble, but it works.

A second method requires skin fold calipers. These require that you determine the fat content of the skin by taking a 'pinch" at various places with large calipers that give you the thickness of the "pinches" and consequently an estimate of the fat content. This can easily be performed by a nurse or even by you. The calipers come in a kit that, along with your weight and height measurements, gives you a good estimate of your body fat. You can modify this by getting a friend to pinch you at various places and estimate the space between the fingers. Grab between your thumb and forefinger and estimate the thickness. Ideally, it would be about one half inch. If it's an inch or more, you're definitely overweight. But, there's a third method that is even better. I call it the paper bag method.

Paper Bag Method

For this method you'll need a paper bag with holes cut so you can see out of them when it's put over your head. You can draw a face on it if you wish. You'll need a tape measure, a bathroom scale, and a private room with a mirror sufficiently large to see your entire body.

First obtain your nude weight, then take the bag and tape into the room, close the door, and be sure you'll be alone. Strip to the minimum (nude if possible), put the bag over your head, and make the following evaluations.

Take a long, slow look at your body. Do you have a slender build? Long or short legs? Are your hips and chest about the same width? Can you see "rolls" around the waist? Do you have a "gut" or are you slender in the stomach? I'm asking you to look at yourself without seeing your face. I want you to see your body as other people do. Are you slender or are you fat or do you have a build that's somewhat beefy without being fat? I'm asking you to be realistic about your own body. Decide whether you're fit or fat.

First look at your neck and ankles. Answer two questions. "Do you have fat ankles and a short neck, or even no neck? If you do, you're an "endomorph" or a "brachiotype"; that means you'd be more likely to be large in frame and to be beefy. In short, if your ankles and neck are not slender, there's a good chance you'll not be slender.

Now look at your knees with your feet together. You should see definite cracks of light above and below your knees. If you don't, you've got a lot of work to do, because you should get your weight down so that the light shines through.

Place your hands at the middle of your hips. Is there about an inch of flesh over the bones? That's about how much should be there. If it's more, especially a lot more, you've got serious weight to lose.

Now measure your hips and your waist. Your waist divided by your hips should be about 0.9 for men and 0.8 for women. When those ratios increase, especially above one, the risk of heart disease increases dramatically.

Measure at mid-chest. For men, this should be about equal to or greater than hips. For women, under the breasts, the same rule holds. If the hips are greater, you're pear shape and that's no good. You've got two tasks; take weight off the hips and build the chest.

Turn sideways, stand straight, and examine your buttocks and your stomach. Without turning green from holding your breath, you should have a slight turning in just below your rib cage so your stomach is flat. However, if you decided honestly that you don't have a neck, have fat ankles, and short legs, you might not have the slight indentation below your rib cage, but your abdomen should still be flat.

Study after study has confirmed that the "paunch" seen on so many men is a warning of possible heart disease, and it is definitely associated with high blood pressure. Abdominal fat is the easiest fat to put on, and the most difficult to take off. If you're a man and you look even slightly pregnant, you're fat. Women sometimes get a bulge as a result of having children. A bulge in older women can develop from extreme osteoporosis where the spine actually compresses and the abdomen bulges because it's somewhat compressed. This is rare, however. In just about every case, it's the remnants of childbirth and it can be worked into shape. Everyone should be able to get his or her stomach flattened from the side view.

Still looking sideways, tighten your buttocks. See if they are either flat or rounded, but not hanging down. Are they hard? You've probably got buttocks, but you don't want it to be flab.

After all this, decide whether you should lose some weight. If you're seriously overweight, you knew it before you started looking at yourself objectively. On the other hand, if you're just a little overweight, decide how much you should lose. Go climb on the scale and set a target.

Suppose you want to get 10 pounds off. It shouldn't surprise you that 60% of Americans at one time or another, in any given year, go on a diet, and that 49% of people between 35 and 50 alone want to lose from 5 to 10 pounds and have a great deal of difficulty doing it. Since you've got high blood pressure, it's essential that you get your weight back to normal; it wouldn't hurt to be a little underweight.

Origins of Overweight

Excess weight is the result of eating more food than you burn. Your body is designed (or evolved) to survive in a world of scarcity. So, when there's an excess available, it's very good at storing those extra calories as fat. Fat, consider that stick of butter, is an excellent form of storage for calories. It conserves 9 calories per gram; that's about 3,500 calories for each pound, and it's pliable at body temperature and requires no water for storage—it's anhydrous.

Carbohydrate, consider starch or sugar, is solid at room temperature and must be dissolved in water to be used by the body. In fact, for every pound of carbohydrate, the body would require three pounds of water. Therefore, in contrast to fat, carbohydrate is "hydrated," and one pound, yielding 1,800 calories, is really four pounds of total weight—that's 1,800 calories for four pounds or only 450 calories per pound in contrast to fat at 3,500 calories per pound. And, if the Creator had decided to store extra calories as carbohydrate, all the extra water would cause elevated blood pressure. Now you know why the body stores its reserve calories as fat—it's simply more efficient. We're fortunate that extra calories are stored as fat, and not as carbohydrate. The problem is why we get fat in the first place.

Heredity and Excess Fat

Excess weight comes from consuming more calories than we burn. That's the basic science of the story, but some issues need to be dealt with. There seem to be several reasons why some people are heavier than others on seemingly the same food intake.

First, the majority of our daily calorie expenditure is for basal metabolism. That's the energy we would expend just to keep our body going if we stayed in bed all day. Some people have a lower basal metabolism than others, and it's lowest in overweight people. Their extra fat acts as an insulator, so they don't lose as much heat to the environment, for example.

Second, there's a current concept called the "set point" theory. This concept teaches that there's a percentage of body fat that gets deeply rooted in our brain early in life and the body "eats" to maintain that level. Only by working at this set point can we establish a lower, healthier weight.

Third, or perhaps as part of the first two concepts, the cell size, cell number hypothesis emerged. In this concept, the small child, during the first two years, develops more cells for the storage of fat. In a sense, it's as though the child develops a large number of balloons to carry through life. In contrast, some infants don't carry large numbers of fat cells (balloons), but the ones they have can become enormous.

So, if we combine all these concepts, we conclude that some people develop a high "set point" that gives them a certain fat level; and they store fat either as lots of small fat cells or as fewer, but larger fat cells. Either system of storing fat actually makes it easier or harder for the plastic surgeon who devotes his practice to removing fat. Some types of fat are more like an appendage and easy to suck out; other types of fat are inside the lean muscle tissue and are extremely dangerous to remove.

Weight loss is the same no matter what the storage form and no matter what the "set point." You've got to burn more calories than you consume and keep doing that for a long time. Exercise is the only thing we know that will produce lean muscle.

Weight Loss Arithmetic

Suppose you've got to drop a total of 10 pounds of fat. At 3,500 calories per pound, that means you've got to create a deficit of 35,000 calories. You can develop a daily caloric expenditure of 2,200 calories if you're a woman and 2,500 if you're a man. And while you can consume very few calories, even starve, for a day or two, you can't do it for a prolonged period. So, let's look at what we can do on average.

On average, if you follow the plan I'll give you in a few pages, you'll consume 1,000 to 1,200 calories daily for a long period of time. Well, 2,200 minus 1,000 leaves a daily deficit of 1,200. That means you'll lose one pound every three days if you're true to yourself. Or, put another way, it'll take 30 days to lose the 10 pounds.

The weight doesn't come off steadily, though. First, you'll drop some stored carbohydrate and extra salt. That means a big water loss. In fact, I've seen many people lose 5% of body weight in the first five days. But lost carbohydrate and its water will be restored by your body even while you're still losing weight. People who regain water and carbohydrate weight while they're actually losing fat often despair because they seem to gain weight. I assure you, they were actually losing weight, because in the clinic we could precisely measure the fat loss and it would be declining.

Follow the plan I give you and you'll lose weight. There will be times when you seem to gain weight. But, if you're true to yourself and stick with your program, you can bring off 1½ to 2 pounds each week over a long period of time and gain a whole new outlook on life.

Can I Lose It Faster?

A woman weighing 150 pounds should not lose more than 1½ to 2 pounds per week steadily. A larger man, say 195 to 225, can proportionately lose more because he's larger.

It's not only unsafe to do it more rapidly, but also impossible. I'll do some arithmetic.

Suppose you're trying to drop 10 pounds. That's a 35,000-calorie loss, and the 1,000-calorie plan I set up creates a daily deficit of 1,200 calories. Let's just suppose you go a step further and consume only 500 calories daily. That creates a daily deficit of 1,700 calories. If you could keep it up, your weight loss would occur in 20 days. Sound pretty good? It's actually pretty grim. Eating 500 calories daily is unsafe unless your health is carefully monitored by a doctor. And the calorie count is so low that it requires the exclusive use of formulated foods that you simply drink. I'll explain how to use those weight-loss drinks, but in a sensible way. You can use them for a day or two, some people even three or four, but then you'll need food. Also, you've got to learn to eat correctly, and you don't do that by drinking some sort of "mulch" for quick loss. Believe me, there's no simple way to take the weight off. A 1,000-calorie diet will do it very nicely. It's safe and you'll be training yourself to eat for the new you.

Set Point Deception

Do you get the nagging feeling that your "set point" will slowly make you regain all that weight? Many people have used it as an excuse, and I know of one person, a nurse, who gives lectures to that effect. In fact, the "set point" is not fact—it's theory. Keeping weight off once lost requires willpower—tremendous willpower—and no matter how sophisticated the reasons scientists give for regaining weight, it remains a matter of will power.

But amid all the scientific rhetoric, there is experimental evidence to show that if a "set point" exists, it slowly adjusts to your new body weight. That's good news and bad news. Good news because if you lose weight and keep it off, your body will eventually accept the new weight as "normal" with its new "set point." Bad news if you get overweight, because it'll do the same thing in the wrong direction and accept serious overweight as the "set point."

With all this talk of "set point" and "fat cell" numbers, you can become addled. Just look at it this way. Your body adapts, but it takes time. You are going to get your weight and your blood pressure into line and your body will adapt to the new you. But you must take the responsibility and make it happen and before long, it will be normal not to be overweight and to have normal blood pressure.

Dieting for Weight Loss

Dieting for weight loss is simple in principle: All you've got to do is reduce your caloric intake to 1,000 calories daily, carry out a normal routine, get about 200 to 250 calories of exercise, and you've done it! That's a mouthful, and we'll do it a step at a time. Also, there's an entire chapter on exercise.

Start by using some rules that are absolutely proven to aid dieting. They also help you develop a new way of life, so the weight stays off. These rules have been identified by the experts over many years. More important, they have been refined by people who have lost weight using them.

Rule 1.   Food Diary. Keep an accurate food diary and write a critique in it at the end of each day. Don't omit a single morsel.

Rule 2.   Bulk at Each Meal. Salads, fruits, cereals, grains, and vegetables can be used in unlimited abundance. Every meal should include a vegetable, grain, or salad. Eating for bulk is common sense eating. Compare a pat of butter (about one ounce), which contains 250 calories, to a head of lettuce or a large apple, which contains up to 150 calories. Throw in a large carrot for another 100 calories. You can swallow an ounce of butter without chewing, but not the apple, lettuce, or carrot. That's what bulk is all about.

Rule 3. Avoid Red Meat. Don't eat red meat; eat fish and poultry (skin removed) barbecued or broiled.

Rule 4. Eat Starchy Foods. Eat things such as rice, baked potato (no butter or sour cream), or pasta (plain tomato sauce). Always eat a single serving.

Rule 5. Eat All the Green Salad You Want. Snack on raw vegetables and popcorn with no butter or salt.

Rule 6. Fruit for Dessert. If you must eat dessert, make it fresh fruit, an apple, pear, orange, or grapefruit.

Rule 7. Alcohol. No alcoholic beverages!

Rule 8. Purchase a book that gives calories, sodium, and potassium. A number have been identified at the end of this chapter. I strongly urge you to obtain *Food Values* by Pennington and Church.

Rule 9. Fat Bag. Every time you lose a pound of weight, put a pound of sand (pet supply store) in a cloth bag. Put it in a prominent place; if you regain a pound, remove it from the bag. Start a new bag every 10 pounds.

Rule 10. Sodium. Limit each meal to 200 milligrams of sodium and strive for a K Factor of 3 or more.

Rule 11. Potassium. Be sure to get 3,000 milligrams daily. If in doubt, use a little salt substitute (preferably not potassium chloride) at mealtime.

Meals

The object is to eat two meals of about 200 to 250 calories each; then have one 500- to 600-calorie meal each day. You can socialize that way, and a 600-calorie meal can be quite effective eating.

In Chapter Thirteen, you already have some meals that are completely acceptable. Consider the following day, which leaves room for many other options. With a little effort, you can find many foods to eat.

Basic Breakfast	225 calories
Luncheon Salad, no dressing, with half serving of tuna chunks	220 calories
Dinner of chicken breast, baked potato, with 1 tablespoon sour cream, and broccoli	400 calories
Daily total	825 calories
Dessert, melon	33 calories
Snack, apple	80 calories

Dietary Drinks

These products are often criticized and never applauded. In my opinion, they can be used effectively and make life convenient. I cite two that I know of and urge you to seek others. Before using these products, I urge you to carefully evaluate the nutrition label. You may want to read about them in *The Food Book*. Too many of them contain too much sodium and lots of sugar. And sugar works against any diet, especially if you have high blood pressure. Many them (e.g., Slim Fast) are so low in calories as to require monitoring by a doctor or registered dietician.

Shaklee Products

Meal Shakes: Prepared with skim milk, provide 230 calories, 200 milligrams of sodium, and 650 of potassium. If made with low-sodium reconstituted dry milk, the sodium is about 100.

Carnation Products

Breakfast Bars: When used as a meal substitute, they provide 200 calories and 185 milligrams of sodium. Both within the safe range.

Supplements—Insurance

In Chapter Twelve I identified a comprehensive supplement. Whenever you are restricting your caloric intake, you should take a supplement as a nutrition insurance policy. Although you will hear from many doctors, dieticians, and nutritionists that you can get all you need from your food, believe me when I say you cannot. Indeed, a recent survey showed that 55% to 60% of registered dieticians used supplements regularly. These are the same people who say you can get along without them. In the real world you can't. Ask them why they use supplements when they say that.

Exercise

Chapter Sixteen is about exercise. It tells you how much you need regularly and why. For anyone on a weight-loss diet, 250 calories of exercise daily is an essential ingredient. It can be done by walking or any of a variety of activities. The important thing is that exercise helps to shift weight from inert fat to more active "red" tissue. This increases your basal metabolism, helps accelerate weight loss, and helps you develop more lean body mass.

Food Diaries and Fat Bags

I have never met a person who doesn't benefit from or need some positive feedback. Positive feedback is like food for the ego; it's a pat on the back. Unfortunately, losing weight or reducing blood pressure is like writing . . . it's lonely. So, sometimes you've got to be your own best friend and that means monitoring progress.

If you've started a food diary, you should be keeping track of your improved food habits, your blood pressure, and pulse. Now take note of your weight or waist measurement. You'll learn to take some satisfaction in saying, "I did that!" But I like another device I mentioned in the rules: the Fat Bag.

A Fat Bag sounds like a gimmick, until you've filled one. It's a cloth bag (actually paper will do, if it's strong) into which you put a pound of sand (found at pet supply stores) or sugar every time you lose a pound of weight. At ten pounds, start a second bag, and so on. These bags serve a second purpose. Pick them up and carry them around for a while sometime. Then think to yourself how much your heart had to pump to push blood through all that flab. Give yourself a medal; you've earned it!

Summary

It is absolutely essential that you do a personal assessment to see if you are fit or fat. Strive to get your body into shape so your general assessment is realistic and you can pass the bag test with an "I'm satisfied!" If you need to lose some weight, diet sensibly and maintain your sodium–potassium balance at the same time. Set realistic goals; use a food diary and fat bag to know where you're going and how you're getting there.

Nutrition insurance is essential when you're dieting.

Additional Reading

Fit or Fat?
Bailey, Covert
Houghton Mifflin, 1978

The Fit or Fat Target Diet
Bailey, Covert
Houghton Mifflin, 1984

The Pritikin Permanent Weight-Loss Manual
Pritikin, Nathan
Bantam Books, 1985

Chapter Sixteen

Exercise

Success Loves Company

A recent study proved a point about success in exercise programs. It proved that success loves company. The most successful adults, by about 50%, were those who exercised as a husband-and-wife team. Most people who approach it with a spouse or close friend succeed. The marriage vows say "for better or for worse"; they should add "with aerobics."

Exercise Helps

Moderate regular exercise improves cardiac output, reduces blood pressure, and increases lean body mass. Many studies have shown that regular exercise, for six or more months, reduces blood pressure by about 9%. That's a lot of information and it's worth looking at it a step at a time.

Improved cardiac output (think back to Chapter One) means the heart pumps more blood with each beat. In other words, regular exercise improves the pumping efficiency of the heart—it makes your heart a stronger muscle. Now that shouldn't surprise you; after all, the heart is a muscle, and how do you improve the strength and flexibility of any muscle? Exercise, that's how! So, regular moderate exercise will improve the muscles being used in the exercise . . . including the heart. Every study confirms that the exercise must be done regularly and steadily. Regularly means about five times weekly or more and steadily means that the effects of this activity start to be obvious in about a month, are really clear in six months, and after a year there's no comparison to the starting point.

Moderate means that it has to be vigorous enough and long enough each time to have an effect—you need to sweat a little—but not so vigorous that you are constantly sore, tired, or exhausted. That translates to vigorous walking for about 40 to 50 minutes daily or jogging 20 to 30 minutes. There are many other forms of exercise that work as well or better and we'll explore them as alternatives.

When I say exercise reduces blood pressure by about 9%, that's an average. In a recent study reported in the *Journal of the American Medical Association*, the reduction reported amounted to 13% or more in some individuals, but on the average was about 9%. You can do some quick arithmetic to see that that reduction will take some people from the "high blood pressure" category to the "high normal category," and with the dietary effort described in this book, they're home free as the saying goes. But remember the old caveats. You've got to do it regularly and it takes time for the results to become apparent.

Now, after saying all that, I want to remind you of something. Most adults who own running shoes only use them once a week for their intended purpose. Put another way: "The road to hell is paved with good intentions." Don't add paving stones to that road.

Unexpected Benefits

Exercise is synergistic. Synergism, from the Greeks, means the sum is greater than its parts. Simply put, if you add the benefits of exercise to your dietary program, you get something even greater than you would have imagined. Satisfaction comes with accomplishment; we humans respond to positive reinforcement. You will begin to find satisfaction as you gain flexibility, shift fat to muscle, and can perform tasks you had once thought hopeless. But that's no different than doing anything well.

Mental alertness always improves with physical fitness because improved muscle tone brings improved circulation. It follows that improved circulation brings more oxygen and nourishment to your master organ, the brain.

Sleep will be sounder, but not because you are tired; on the contrary, you will have more energy. You sleep better because everything about your body is more efficient. And although the restrictive power of sound sleep remains a scientific mystery, no one can ever doubt its miraculous mental and physical value.

Regularity of bowel function will improve, another of the synergistic benefits of exercise with dietary commitment. Although dietary fiber improves regularity and bowel function, the regularity of exercise, which tones all muscles, including those of the bowel, helps them to respond easily and regularly.

Bone strength will also increase. A national epidemic of osteoporosis is sweeping the United States. Osteoporosis is a decline in bone density due in large part to inadequate dietary calcium and exercise in the childhood and adolescent years. Once women are past menopause, hormonal changes bring about an acceleration of bone loss, so the problem is even more critical. Two factors require personal control—dietary calcium and exercise. This dietary plan will take care of the calcium, but only you can take care of the exercise.

Can You Do It?

No one is so unfit, so overweight, so physically handicapped that he or she can't exercise. I have had the beautiful experience of seeing 81-year-old women start an exercise program to help their arthritis. My own mother, at 82, mounts a stationary bicycle each day and peddles for 10 to 20 minutes. Now, if she can do it, so can you.

I have run so many 10K races against wheelchair athletes, blind runners, or runners with arms missing that I no longer accept physical handicap as an excuse. There's an exercise available to everyone just as there are excuses available to everyone. It's too bad that the two easiest forms of exercise are running from personal responsibility and jumping to conclusions.

"But, Dr. Scala, I don't have time." Baloney! Nothing is as important as your health, but nothing is so easily avoided or procrastinated as changing health habits. You'll just have to get up earlier, change your eating pattern, or stop work earlier. But the time exists.

"It's dark and dangerous in the early morning or early evening!" No excuse! The plethora of excellent indoor exercise devices available nowadays that have been tested and proven effective make it possible to never go outside. I'll identify some of them for you.

I'll make a proposition. One of the benefits of regular exercise is that you'll require less sleep. So, if you get up earlier, it'll become habit and you'll never miss the time. Time can be found if you want it!

"But Dr. Scala, I'm so out of shape it'll take too long." Look it doesn't take as long to get into shape as it took to get out. Furthermore, you should start slowly and work up. Indeed, a good start is to walk 30 minutes at a vigorous pace each day. That doesn't even require special shoes, except ones that won't cause blisters. Then, work up to 50 minutes and you're on your way.

Consult Your Doctor

By all means discuss exercise with your doctor. Before anyone with high blood pressure starts an exercise program, they should get the go ahead. Ask your doctor if it's okay for you to start a moderate aerobic exercise program. Explain that you're going to start slowly, for example, a walking program, and work up to something more active. The doctor will explain any restrictions, but it's a rare doctor who will say no to vigorous walking unless your condition is exceptionally serious. And then ask if you can walk slowly for 10 minutes and rest for 5, etc. There's an exercise program for everyone; you've simply got to find yours.

Ideal Exercise

Maximum heart rate is the beats per minute that is the upper limit you should achieve for your age. It's a rate that most doctors won't allow you to achieve during an exercise physical unless they must for some specific technical purpose. You can easily determine yours—just subtract your age from 220 to get your maximum. Then take 70% of that number and you've got the training heart rate (THR) you should strive for in exercising. An ideal exercise will get your heart rate (pulse) to that figure and maintain it for 20 to 30 minutes. Notice the emphasis is on pulse rate and not on the form of exercise. That simply confirms my point that there are unlimited exercise variations available.

By exercising for 20 minutes three or more times weekly, you achieve a training effect. A training effect stresses the cardiovascular system sufficiently so it responds by slowly building more capacity. In the long run, the heart pumps more efficiently, more capillaries develop and the muscles around the arteries become stronger. The magic of 70% of maximum heart rate and 20 minutes is that it's a sort of optimum.

I'm writing this at age 53, so my maximum is $220-53 = 167$. And my THR is 70% of 167, or 117. So I should exercise vigorously enough to get my heart beating within 10% of my THR; that's from about 110 to 123. Starting out, stay at the low end, and once you're about 6 to 12 months along, go nearer the high end.

You should not go more than 70% of maximum level—
the THR—unless a physician approves or recommends it.
You can stay below 70%, however, if you extend the exercise time. For example, 20 minutes of jogging at 70%
equals about 50 minutes of vigorous walking at 50%. You
can achieve a training effect by simply putting more time
into a lower level of activity.

I urge you to purchase one of the books I have identified
at the end of this chapter for more thorough exercise programs and an explanation of the heart rate objectives.

How Important Is the THR?

Any time someone gives you such precise instructions,
recognize that it's an average and you should probably fall
somewhere within the range. As varied as we humans are
in appearance, so do we vary right down to each of the 50
trillion (50 with 13 zeros) cells that make up the average
150-pound person. And this variation extends to our training needs as well; but if you start an exercise program that
your doctor says is okay for you, you should be able to
achieve your normal THR after a month or two. Most
people fit in the normal range.

Suppose you start with a resting pulse of about 80 or
more? Then, you'll reach your THR more quickly and have
to be more moderate than others. But, as you become
more fit, your resting pulse will be lower. For example, my
normal resting pulse is 54 and I can't get to my THR unless
I really work hard; in contrast, I have friends whose resting
pulse is 75 to 80, who reach THR quickly and easily.

Suppose you can't exercise fast enough to get to THR.
For example, you're truly out of shape or have a heart
problem that prohibits it. No problem! The THR is an
objective that makes it easier because, if exercise is done at
THR for 20 minutes, 3 to 5 times weekly, it achieves the
training effect. It's a kind of "optimum" between time
spent and level of activity. You can get the same result at a
lower level of activity for a longer period of time.

For example, suppose you can get about halfway to THR from your resting pulse. That's okay. Simply do it about 2½ times as long. So, instead of jogging 20 minutes, walk for 50 minutes. It's that simple. I emphasize 2½ times because the trade-off is not direct. A little more time is required at the less vigorous level, but the result is the same.

Exercise Programs

I urge people to start a walking program. Walking is easy, doesn't require anything special, and you get to see things along the way. Just don't stop and talk. Many other variations of exercise are also excellent. As long as they get you to your THR, and you can sustain them for 20 minutes or more, they are fine. That opens up many opportunities. Take a look at some of them.

Individual Exercise

Walking (can also be done with weights)
Jogging
Cycling (on road or stationary bike)
Swimming
Aerobics (low and high impact)
Rowing (boat or machine)
Cross-country skiing (real or simulated)
Step climbing (real or simulated)
Skating (ice and roller)
Jazzercise (also called Dancersize)

Sports

Tennis if it's vigorous
Racquetball
Handball

Waterpolo
Basketball
Hockey

Notice I've left out golf and weight lifting and specified that tennis should be vigorous. The reasons for these restrictions illustrate what you're trying to accomplish and it's worth reviewing again.

Golf is a great way to ruin a walk. You walk a little, stop to plan your next shot, etc., wait for others to hit, etc. That's not steady exercise even though it takes the better part of a complete day. It may be excellent recreation, but it's not the way to obtain a training effect.

Anaerobic exercise like weight lifting or short-distance running may add muscle mass, but it doesn't improve aerobic capacity. That is, it doesn't cause the heart to achieve its THR and remain there for 20 minutes or more. Tennis usually fits this criterion because of so many frequent stops for most amateurs. If, however, you play tennis vigorously for a long time (many sets), and don't stop and talk, it will produce a training effect. One advantage is that you'll get good at one of the world's greatest social games and get in shape as well.

Ideal Total Exercise

Many joggers and cyclists feel the effects of fitness and become dedicated. Indeed, they often start slowly and before long the runners enter 10K races and cyclists start with century runs. And believe me, I've had many pupils do this with fantastic results; I'm proud of them. But when people ask me what I do, I always talk about my total program that starts with simulated cross-country skiing. Let me make my point.

Jogging and cycling are excellent for cardiovascular purposes. But have you ever noticed, for example, that their shoulders often diminish, and especially for cyclists, their legs get very large. It's because the body adapts. And if you jog, you need large muscle mass in your legs, but not in the shoulders; similar for cycling. The same but opposite effect unavoidably occurs in the wheelchair "runner" whose shoulders and arms become very well developed.

All this is why I'm a fan of simulated cross-country skiing. This program uses a device that exercises both upper and lower body. It uses both arms and legs and consequently requires a little bit of time to get coordinated. The training effect is excellent, however, and generally improves both upper and lower muscle masses. Consequently, the shoulders, arms, hips, and legs become conditioned at the same time. An added benefit is derived from the twisting effect in cross-country skiing. It comes from moving the left arm, right leg and vice versa. The benefit is to help reduce the fat pads that so many adults develop around the hips . . . they're called "love handles."

In addition to 20 to 40 minutes of cross-country skiing, a few other exercises are essential to help improve "lean body mass" and general conditioning. I identify them as stretching and toning.

Stretch

Before exercising, some stretching exercises are essential. Stretching is simple but essential, since it helps to prevent soreness and injury. Common sense will tell you what to do.

I can't emphasize enough the need to take all exercise seriously. There are many fine, well-written books on the subject. Although I favor the books by Kenneth Cooper of the Aerobics Institute, any of those listed at the end of this chapter are excellent. I urge you to select one you find easy to follow.

Stretching the calf muscles and Achilles tendons of the legs is easily accomplished by simply attempting to touch the toes while holding the feet flat on the ground. A good variation is to cross the feet. Don't bounce up and down in an attempt to get closer to the toes; that can hurt. A variation is to face and reach to a wall and stagger your feet, bending the forward knee with the rear foot flat on the ground.

Hamstrings of the upper leg are easily stretched by two methods. I like to raise one leg about hip high (no higher) on a fence or other support, and while holding it there, stretch my arms to touch the toes of that foot. Don't bounce in an attempt to reach the toes; a long slow stretch is best. Alternatively, straddle your legs, facing forward with chest over your left knee and arms clasped behind your back. Now slowly straighten your legs. Reverse it with your chest over the right knee.

Hip stretches are easily done by placing one knee on the floor with the other knee over the toes of that leg so you're kneeling on one knee with your back straight; then lean as far forward on the upright knee as possible, holding the other knee and foot in position on the floor.

Lower back stretching is essential, especially as people get older. Back stretches are accomplished by lying flat on the back, pulling one knee at a time to the chest, and holding it for about 20 to 30 seconds. After doing each leg about 5 to 10 times, do both legs together and hold for 30 or more seconds.

Tone

Toning exercises give tone to your muscle groups: for example, a flat stomach, thin thighs, hips without love handles, a firm derrier instead of a soft fat derrier, and tight arm muscles instead of soft hanging flab. Obviously these are important to help the new you gain a better appearance. One reason I recommend simulated cross-country skiing is that it does the arms, hips, and thighs at one time. If that's not your program, and even if it is, there are exercises that help tone. Please, however, be sure to purchase one of the books at the end of this chapter.

Sit-ups with knees bent will, in the long run, flatten the tummy. But they take time to be effective, so perseverance pays. If you're one of those women who cannot do a complete sit-up (often the price for children), there are devices you can purchase that will provide support. Alternatively, get in position and simply lift your head as high as possible each time. Slowly you will get better as your tummy muscles flatten and strengthen. Whatever type you do, work up to about 30 daily and do them daily. You will eventually notice a flattening of your stomach and a reduction in hip circumference.

Love handles are dealt with by taking weight, about 10 pounds of books, for example, holding it hip high in front with both hands, feet about 12 inches apart, and rotating slowly as far as possible to each side and holding for about 10 seconds. Work up to 30 on each side daily and eventually the love handles will firm and disappear. Perseverance is essential.

Thighs are thinned by lying on the side and doing alternate leg raises with each leg held straight. Start slowly as these can make you stiff and sore, but work up to about 20 for each leg. Once more, perseverance is required, but results will slowly appear.

Arms are firmed by doing work. Now's the time for those little weights you see people swing as they walk. You don't have to purchase anything sophisticated; anything that's convenient will do. Simply hold your elbow at the body and lift the weight up slowly and down slowly. Remember, the weight need not be heavy, just do the exercise regularly. You can do this while walking or, if you're good, while jogging.

Television Stretching

If you are up to it, there are daily TV exercise programs that emphasize stretching and limbering. Many of them are quite advanced and you simply cannot keep up. But get the motion down properly and go at your own pace. Remember, you are not expected to keep up with or exceed what they are doing; rather, your pace is determined by your own body. Recently, videotapes of slow-paced exercise have become available.

Don't Do Anaerobic Exercise

Throughout this discussion, I have emphasized walking, running, swimming, and cross-country skiing, done for at least 20 minutes and up to an hour daily. These are all called aerobic exercises because they involve prolonged use of the cardiovascular system to move large amounts of oxygen in the blood to the entire body. I said they produce a training effect; that's another way of saying they tone the entire cardiovascular system.

Anaerobic exercise, in contrast, doesn't rely on prolonged use of the cardiovascular system. As the name implies, it's exercise done for short periods; it does not rely on prolonged cardiovascular activity. Good examples of anaerobic activities are weight lifting, some track events like shot put or discus throw, short dashes, and everyday activities like running for the bus or train.

Obviously, there are times when running for buses or trains is unavoidable, but other anaerobics can and should be avoided. They should be avoided because they elevate the blood pressure and when done regularly for a long period of time, have a permanent effect. Avoiding anaerobic exercise eliminates weight lifting, short "dash" type running, and similar activities, including a fast 50-yard swim. You know these types of exercise don't help because they create an oxygen debt that has you gasping for breath when you stop. If you can't do it for at least 20 minutes, then don't do it at all.

Timing: Exercise and Stress

Think back to Chapter Nine and Colonel Oliver's stressful situation, the racing car drivers, and his type A behavior. In every case, conditioning for stress is important, but so is its relief. Stress is conveniently relieved by exercise because it provides a convenient means of eliminating the excess flood of materials that have spilled into the blood from the stress.

These excesses include hormones, fats, and blood sugars. The origins of stress are what we call the preparation for "fight or flight." In short, the body prepares itself to either stand and fight or to run from the danger. And modern verbal battles don't count. So it follows that if you can take your exercise at the end of the stressful period, you'll benefit more.

In fact, that's what most exercise-stress studies have shown. The example of the race car drivers is one of the best illustrations. The drivers combined the benefits of stress, that is, the preparedness of the hormones, fats, and sugars with the outlet of a hard physical workout for over two hours.

Obviously, we're not all racing car drivers, so we must find other means to relieve the "metabolic potential" that we call the "fight or flight" syndrome.

Aerobic exercises will always be the best vent for stress. That's why I always urge executives to exercise at the end of the day. And since their day is often long, it requires indoor equipment except during long summer evenings.

Alternatively, I know many successful people who put their stressful situations in the morning agenda and use the lunch hour for a 20- or 30-minute jog. Still others will at least take a long uninterrupted walk at lunchtime. If you're in a situation where you can't exercise in the evening or at noon, a morning session will still have many, many benefits. It will condition your body and your cardiovascular system will be able to deal with the stresses of everyday business more effectively. And that's what the next chapter is all about.

Additional Reading

Aerobic Walking
Meyers, Casey
Vintage Books, 1987

Running Without Fear
Cooper, Kenneth H., M.D.
Bantam Books, 1986

Swim for the Health of It
Maglischo, Ernest W. and Brennan, Cathy Ferguson
Mayfield Publishing, 1985

The Aerobics Program for Total Well-Being
Cooper, Kenneth H., M.D.
Bantam Books, 1982

The Complete Book of Exercise Walking
Yanker, Gary D.
Contemporary Books, 1983

The Runner's Handbook
Glover, Bob and Shepherd, Jack
Penguin Books, 1987

Chapter Seventeen

Coping With Stress

White Coat Hypertension

A recent article in the *Journal of the American Medical Association* described "white coat hypertension" as very mild high blood pressure that exists only in the doctor's office. The tenseness that develops when the man or woman in the white coat wraps the cuff around your arm, puts the iced stethoscope to your arm, and says, "Breath normally," can elevate blood pressure. In fact, one estimate says it accounts for one fifth of most mild hypertension. It's just one reason why I urge you to take your own blood pressure regularly.

But the lesson of white coat hypertension is that tenseness elevates blood pressure. And that's as nature intended. It goes back to the fight or flight syndrome. When we're threatened our body prepares for fight or flight. That means we need to be sure enough blood goes to the brain so there's plenty of energy to think. Also, it insures that metabolic energy is used for defense and not lost to the atmosphere so peripheral circulation is restricted. It has the added advantage of conserving body fluid, and even urine production slows down.

External Stress

The stress of being examined by a doctor creates sufficient tenseness to elevate the blood pressure to serious levels in some people. We call these people stress-sensitive individuals, since they respond to even mild stress with elevated blood pressure.

Two questions are obvious. Why would they respond to something as nonthreatening as the doctor? How do they control themselves so that doesn't happen? We can immediately see two approaches: Learn to understand which events are threatening, and develop a plan of coping and a lifestyle that helps your body relax. Let's go at them one at a time.

What Is Threatening?

I love to work with children of alcoholics because alcoholics have a beautiful prayer: Lord, help me to recognize those things I cannot change from those things I can change and grant me the wisdom to know the difference.

Many things in life threaten our equilibrium. These usually appear in the world of work, but they also appear in our home life. For example, in work you can easily be trapped in a position that affords no upward mobility. In short, you're trapped and possibly faced with many pressures. Pressure can range from an insensitive boss to being passed by for promotion and placed under someone who is your junior, or having unreasonable work deadlines or demands placed upon you.

In the home a myriad of things can threaten equilibrium. A study conducted by the University of California at Berkeley of things that caused the greatest hassles in home life turned up an unsuspected finding. Most people's lives were hassled by their pets. It was a surprising finding, because the family pet is not a necessity; it's an option. Other problems range from an alcoholic spouse to excessive demands for more time to do church work. Common sense dictates what needs to be done.

First, assess what can be changed from what cannot. In my management career I often suggested to employees that they develop a good resume and see what opportunities were available for them. This proposal had two eventualities. One was for the employee to realize how great it was for his career to remain in my employ; the other was to recognize that better opportunities existed and the difficulty was in choosing. Either way, as a result, I had an employee who knew where he stood. Then he and I could deal with his work situation so he wouldn't expect a promotion that didn't exist. And if his personal circumstances justified it, he'd take another job. We all came out on top, because the environment was open. My first lesson is to open up your life and identify clearly that which you can change and that which you cannot change. Now, how do you cope with that which you cannot change?

Oriental Ninjitsu martial arts philosophy teaches, "Run toward the danger." Most people who threaten expect us to run away . . . after all, that's why they threaten. So the first step is to confront the threat, "run toward the danger," and, for example, either decide that the work situation is fair or not fair. If not fair, identify the source and deal with it appropriately. Recognize that soft-spoken compliments and positive reinforcement produce better results than caustic comments and negative reinforcement. Positive reinforcement is a selfish attitude because it's designed to produce personally favorable results. In contrast, caustic comments and negative reinforcement usually become more stressful to the person making them than to the person to whom they are directed. Let me give an illustration.

Positive Reinforcement

In my past work environment, my boss made it quite obvious that he didn't feel comfortable with me. I was left out of important meetings, conveniently omitted from luncheon lists, and reports from my network of friends indicated that most of his comments about me were negative. The situation was very stressful until I recognized what I could accomplish.

I made an assessment of my contributions to the corporate effort. I committed myself to doing them so well and so professionally that no one could criticize their form, substance, or execution. Simultaneously, I decided that whatever my boss did that was positive, I would give him what I call a "thumbs-up."

I remember one note very well; he had a luncheon to recognize some five-year employees . . .

> Dear Charles:
> It was kind of you to recognize [some names] for their loyal service. They needed to have someone say "I care" and you did it well.
> Congratulations.
> Respectfully,
> Jim

The reason I remember it well is that it had nothing to do with me. But I knew he had done it, so it was part of my plan. Now, I'm not kidding myself. He didn't start liking me; his ego wouldn't permit that. But I started hearing positive comments from my network. Things like, "Charles said you did a great job in Minneapolis," or "Have you noticed the attendance at Jim's talks?" Lo and behold, one day he previewed a video I had made. I got a note saying it was a good job.

Do you believe the stress in my work environment had decreased? I never got invited to the meetings, the luncheons, etc.; I knew I couldn't change his ego. But, true to the Ninjitsu philosophy, I ran toward the danger and overcame it in the best way: positive reinforcement.

You can do that in every aspect of your daily life. We do it with our children, our friends, everyone. When I like my wife to dress a certain way, I don't say, "Now this is how you must dress," but rather, "You looked fantastic in that blue form-fitting dress." Guess what style she looks at the next time she shops.

Positive reinforcement works with everyone around you and can do more to relieve external stress than any other technique. But there's some things you must do; that is, be scrupulously honest with yourself. And here's where a plain-spoken friend can help. Make an assessment of the situation, write it out, then ask a friend to read it and offer constructive criticism—emphasis is on constructive. Little phrases like, "Help me understand," not, "You're not being clear."

Personal Positive Reinforcement

I once asked a very successful insurance agent what his secret was. His answer in one word, "Guilt!" His trick was to make someone feel guilty and drive them to purchasing his product. "Of course you want your family safe . . ."

A successful Fuller brush salesman made many sales by simply saying to the housewife, "Did you know that your neighbor scrubs the kitchen floor with the same mop as the bathroom floor?" You'd better believe that woman bought a second mop.

We do the same thing to ourselves all the time by creating guilt. This book is an excellent example. I've explained how you can control your blood pressure by diet and lifestyle. And I've given some simple things that are very powerful. Think how simple they are.

- A food diary
- A daily time for exercise
- A food plan emphasizing natural food
- A concept of positive reinforcement

The logic of these things is impeccable and the science is sound. You'll be giving yourself a thumbs-up every time you do them, and if you slide on one or two once in a while, that's okay. As soon as you get back again, you'll feel so good about yourself you'll be that much stronger.

In contrast, you have a conscience, and it will build a bag of guilt for you if you do nothing. People think that doing nothing is easy. It's not. It's the hardest work an intelligent person can take on. It's hard because the heaviest burden we can carry around is the burden of guilt. So, don't add to your stress by doing nothing—start now.

Goal Setting

Maximum positive reinforcement comes from the satisfaction of achieving a goal that was realistically set. Notice that I said "realistically set." Effective goal setting is not an easy task at first, but it becomes easier with practice. Experts have written books on the subject, but I'll try to summarize what I have gleaned from them.

An effective goal should be clear, concise, and a realistic stretch of your abilities. You should easily be able to write it onto a 3 × 5 note card. It should be kept with you personally and also placed where it can be seen by people who must participate, or from whom you require support. The goal should be reducible to a series of milestones that will make it a reality. Let's do an example.

Suppose you've decided that not only will you begin a walking program, but you'd also like to become a jogger and work up to 2 miles in 15 minutes, 4 times weekly in 6 months' time. So the goal is quite clear if you put as a criteria for success that you'll do it 4 times weekly (on average) for 3 consecutive months. Okay, here's your goal on a 3 × 5 card. Say it's January: "I will jog 2 miles daily in 15 minutes on average, 4 times weekly from June 1 through September 1.

Now, it's January and you're not jogging, you're a bit

overweight, and you've got high blood pressure. But you've got 6 months and are otherwise healthy. Some realistic milestones are as follows:

- Walk 50 yards, jog 50 yards for 2 miles through January 15.
- Walk 50 yards, jog 100 yards for 3 miles through January 30.
- Walk 50 yards, jog 150 yards for 3 miles through February 15.
- Jog 1 mile nonstop by February 28.
- Walk ¼ mile, jog 1½ miles, walk ¼ mile by March 15.
- Jog 2 miles by April 15 in less than 18 minutes.
- Average 8 minutes per mile by May 15 for 3 miles.
- June 1, be timed at 7.5 minutes per mile for 2 miles!

The rest is obvious; you only have to keep up the 15-minute 2-mile pace for 3 months. You will have achieved a level of fitness that will make you feel so good about yourself that you'll want to test more aggressive limits. And, by the way, if you're about 40 years old, you'll be in the top 20% level of fitness for your age. And you will have added a few years to your life expectancy.

Notice that in the training schedule I put some 3-mile jogs at 8 minutes per mile. This is what we call physically stressing yourself so you can develop greater endurance. It makes the 2 miles at 15 minutes less of a stretch.

Now, I said to make others aware of the goal. For example, put a 3 × 5 note card on the family bulletin board. In our house, that's the refrigerator. Sound corny? Well, a recent study showed that spousal support for exercise increases the success rate by about 50%. That's right: An actual study showed clearly that if those closest to you are aware of and support your goals, you'll succeed. Everyone needs some support!

Internal Stress: "Type A Behavior"

You know whether or not you're a Type A personality. If you don't, reread Chapter Nine and purchase Dr. Friedman's book, *Type A Behavior and Your Heart*, even if your heart is as sound as gold bullion. The book will help you understand yourself and gain insight into the behavioral changes you must make. Don't get the idea that you're going to convert from Type A to Type B personality, because you're not. If you are more Type A than Type B, your stress is internally generated and you must cope with yourself. I like to call my Type A traits my own free-floating anxiety and deal with them humorously.

Type A behavior can be channeled successfully to produce a reduction in blood pressure. You simply want to redirect some of the energy into activities that will bring about net relaxation of internal stresses. One we've already discussed: exercise.

Exercise for a Type A personality should become sufficiently strenuous that it produces a good sweat. And it should not be done as a competitive effort. In short, if you decide that handball is the way for you to get exercise, then you are likely to increase tension by your inborn overwhelming desire to win and you'll probably lose some friends in the process. Rather, I propose a comprehensive exercise like swimming or cross-country skiing (real or simulated) because it uses the large muscle groups and requires complete physical and mental participation. And, if you absolutely must compete, it's only against yourself.

Relaxation-Diversion

Although I classify exercise as a form of relaxation, in this case I mean relax. Now, relax doesn't mean lie down and sleep. Indeed, it's important to get adequate sleep, but it's just as important to make a substantial effort at an activity that consumes the thoughts but is not stressful. And it's not easy!

It's not easy to relax despite all the devices aimed at efficiency and speed that mark our computer age. The power of technology does not free us for all those things we like. In his book *Time Wars*, Jeremy Rifkin argues that technology seems to bind us even more closely to the grindstone. He says that the inexorable rhythms of the computer are replacing those of natural life. It all boils down to one fact: True relaxation in this high-tech age amounts to hard work.

Hobbies divert, but active hobbies divert most completely and effectively. Active hobbies require physical involvement. Compare furniture making to art collecting.

Furniture making is physical; you've got to saw, measure, plane, sand, hit your thumb a time or two, stain, and perform many tasks that require a great deal of attention. It's not passive at all, but it's not strenuous either; it's complete involvement.

Art collecting requires reading, could involve taking classes, meeting with experts, going to museums and more. But physical activity is not its characterizing element. Surely it requires undivided attention, especially because a lot of money is involved. It can also involve much compulsion. In contrast, furniture making can only move at a certain pace, and it has a factor we'll discuss in Chapter Eighteen— simplicity. Time is required to bring the wood to shape, and your progress is obvious.

Recreation is another means of effective diversion. We enjoy taking Type A personalities on our sailboat. The *La Scala* is a ketch (two masts) and 47 feet overall. It requires attention when sailing, especially in the strong winds of San Francisco Bay or on the Pacific Ocean. Everyone we regard as a Type A has always said, "That's what I need; it takes your complete attention." So I ask them, "What's stopping you?"

I don't suggest that everyone purchase a large sailboat.

Think of all the alternatives, from scuba diving to hang gliding. There's no limit to the opportunities.

Are You Too Old?

I get the "I'm too old" so often that I always stop and remind you that you've never too old. At the local hang gliding school two months ago, the oldest pupil was 74. I had thought I was too old to take up hang gliding and he happened to be flying the day I went to speak to the instructor; another excuse is gone. I didn't do it because I'm chicken!

Meditation

During the 1970s many health scientists were surprised when studies proved conclusively that meditation could produce a reduction in blood pressure. During that period, various types of meditation were being actively pursued on campuses and many other places. I personally know several medical school faculty members who became actively involved and they still use meditation today.

Meditation, done effectively, accomplishes relaxation and diversion. For example, in some Eastern forms of meditation you are given a secret mantra that you continually recite, in an especially relaxed position with your eyes closed, in a quiet place. Your mind is slowly diverted and you enter a trancelike sleep. Your metabolism slows, your blood pressure declines, even your body temperature declines when you are successful. It works.

Other forms of meditation require you to enter the same relaxed position and in your mind's eye visualize a nice, quiet, tranquil scene and slowly let all thoughts flow from your head. When done successfully, it produces the same result.

Meditation works. It can be self-taught, but it works best with some instruction. You can purchase one of the books I have identified to get started. But I urge you, if you're serious, to at least speak to an expert on the subject. You will be pleasantly surprised at how easily it can be done and how effective it can be. Most basic lessons do not require many sessions, and success comes very quickly.

Meditation has an advantage in this fast-paced world we live and work in. All you need is about 20 minutes and a quiet place. No other equipment is required.

Biofeedback

In the beginning of this book, I urged you to purchase a blood pressure measuring device. Now, I want you to use it in a very special way. I want you to experiment in biofeedback.

Biofeedback grew out of the meditation movement and the concept that we have more mental control over our physiology than we might think. Students were hooked up to a pulse meter and told to sit quietly and try to lower their pulse rate. Slowly most of them learned how to do exactly that.

Now, don't expect to sit down and bring your pulse from 80 down to 55; you could probably learn to reduce it from 80 to 72, though. Similarly, by sitting quietly and relaxing, you can probably develop modest blood pressure reduction. It takes perseverance.

Techniques of biofeedback require instruction, or at least a concerted effort. I suggest you start with a book on meditation and learn those techniques before starting a biofeedback program. Either program will produce the same results and are worth the effort.

The Magic Pyramid

Jack, a friend who sees something good in everything that happens, has so amazed me that I had to ask him how it came to be. He credits his mother and tells this story: "I

came home from school with all D's and F's on my report
card. My mother looked at the report card . . . there was
dead silence . . . then she smiled and said, 'Jack I'm so
proud of you.' Amazed, he asked her why, and she replied,'I
know that you don't cheat in school.'

He goes on to tell how it broke the ice, how she motivated him to achieve with his best qualities. They could
then have a productive discussion on his scholastic problems and both move forward.

Growing up in that environment made Jack one of the
most positive people I know. He's had a borderline blood
pressure problem with the constant threat of medication,
complicated by kidney stones. When he asked me if diet
would help, I told him clearly and simply what he had to
do: fundamentally, what's in this book plus the guidelines
he must follow for the kidney stones. His reply was superb.
"Boy, am I glad that I know how far I can go." I laughed
and asked what he meant. He was quick. "I'm lucky; I
know how far I can go with a poor diet, lack of exercise,
and burning the candle at both ends."

There's a major lesson here—a positive attitude can do
everything. I've had surgeon friends talk about patients
who have thrived after serious cancer surgery and others
who have wasted and died. When asked why, their reply is
universal: "Attitude."

Positive thinking can work magic in your life, and for
high blood pressure, I put it at the apex of a pyramid. The
other three base points are exercise, diet, and relaxation.
Diet is the most difficult because we are at the mercy of a
prolific food industry in the land of plenty. The dietary plan
in this book will work, but it will work better if done with
exercise and active relaxation.

Exercise and active relaxation are two activities that must
be done by you yourself. Get guidance, direction, and
advice, but know that no one can do it for you. Set goals,
keep track of your progress, and don't miss any milestones.

Additional Reading

Smart Cookies Don't Crumble
Friedman, Sonya
Pocket Books, 1985

The Joy of Stress
Hanson, Peter J., M.D.
Andrews McMeel and Parker, 1985

Chapter Eighteen

Mental Conditioning

Visualize Success

I once asked a Mexican wood carver in Puerto Vallarta how he could take a piece of drift wood and make it into three whales leaping from the sea. His reply was not unlike that of a child. "God has put the whales in the wood for everyone to see. All I do is cut away the extra." This man doesn't even sketch what he will produce; he simply visualizes it and works the wood until it is finished. He uses two knives, sandpaper, and wax for polishing.

So it is with our lives: What we visualize for ourselves we can become if we hold fast to our vision, strive to achieve it, and let the years come to what they may. This is how some people achieve; they "see" themselves as who they will become and they hold fast to the vision until it is complete.

Health is no different; in fact, it's easier than other goals to visualize and achieve. It simply requires identifying a realistic vision—a goal—and holding on to it and striving until it becomes reality.

The tools are even simpler than the Mexican woodcarver's; common sense, a little reading, and you're fully equipped.

Externalize Your Goals and Success

If you want to regain complete health, to restore normal blood pressure without taking drugs, to eliminate a paunch, to get into shape, then visualize yourself that way. These are realistic goals. Write each objective on a 3 × 5 note card.

The next and very important step is to enlist people around you to support what you are doing. Put your goals out for them to see. In our house, those cards are attached to the refrigerator with magnets.

Don't stop there: Externalize your success. A good example is a Fat Bag for a weight loss objective. Sew one or get someone else to do it, and label it for all the world to see: "Fat Bag!" Place it in a prominent spot so you're aware of your own success and people around you will see how serious you are about your resolve. Keep a running account of blood pressure in your food diary. Jogging, cycling, or tennis scores should be posted next to your goals.

Does this sound corny? It shouldn't! Return with me to the simplicity of the Mexican carver. He visualizes his goal and holds his progress right in his hand all the time. His entire family is there in the same room to support him if he comes onto a tough knot in the wood, to pat him on the back when he succeeds. He doesn't think it's corny for people, especially his loved ones, to see his progress. Why shouldn't you see your progress?

Goal I

Set up a food diary. Actually, this could be called a good-health diary. You should keep a daily record of what, when, why, and where you eat. You should also keep a record of your pulse, blood pressure, and exercise. Then, at the end of the day, write a few sentences, or a paragraph of how well you think you've done.

At first, don't try to use your food diary as a major

vehicle to health; use it to get acquainted with yourself. For example, at the end of the week notice when you eat certain foods and with whom. Look for patterns in your habits that could be improved and write them down; you'll be surprised how they'll disappear.

Goal II

Eat food with a K Factor of at least 3 or 4 that delivers 500 milligrams of sodium daily or less. Write it on 3 × 5 note cards and put one wherever it will help: on the refrigerator, carry one in your pocket, on the dresser, give one to a co-worker. Enlist your doctor's support and accept no less from him or her than support.

Within the framework of your goals you should have one about medication. Don't attempt to get off medication all at once. In fact, that could be dangerous. Rather, in the next chapter you'll see that drug therapy follows progression, and you could easily be on the highest level. That's why you want to enlist your doctor's help and support. Don't accept anything less than support from the doctor. You'll learn that a positive attitude on your part will be contagious.

Goal III

Exercise each day to achieve a reasonable fitness objective. This objective is easy because you know your fitness level. An objective of a 50-minute brisk walk daily for six months might be your best program—but only if you cast it in bronze on a note card and then keep track of your progress. Don't hesitate to join an exercise group or do it with a television program.

Studies have shown time after time that people who exercise with others, especially a spouse, are most successful. There are aerobic groups, walking groups, and cycling groups. I'll bet you can find a "running from responsibility group." But the best is your family. Don't hesitate to take the children out and instill some good health habits at an early age.

Goal IV

Set time aside to smell the roses. Establish time each day for diversion. If it involves your spouse or a friend, it's even better. Make sure it's sufficiently active that it requires your attention, but it doesn't have to be physical. Watching television doesn't count, nor does going to the movies. Joining a theater group could be excellent. A life-long hobby of mine is astronomy and telescope making. So many people have said, "Boy, I wish I had a hobby like that." I simply look at them and tell them they can, right now! But they usually give some excuse like time or something else. Well, one day there's no more time.

Goal V

Practice biofeedback and relaxation. This is the easiest of all objectives, but the one most people don't keep up. I think the reason they don't is because of that complexity the sociologists tell us about. All it requires is about 20 minutes, a quiet place, and you. No special equipment needed. It's best if you can get some instruction or purchase a good book on the subject. You will be amazed at how deceptively simple it is and how effective it can be.

Goal VI

Manage the stress within and without. If you're Type A, use that free-floating anxiety to pursue these goals and that alone will make you succeed. But also manage your external stress. First, identify the sources of stress and go directly toward each one with a program of positive management.

Send a message to each, by example if possible, that makes a statement about how you want to be treated.

I could go on and on about how you should set other objectives that cover other details, but if you can make a significant dent on the above six, you'll gain a longer life with greater abundance. As you progress on these six goals, your self-confidence and self-esteem will increase. You will gain a simplified perspective, like that of the woodcarver of Puerto Vallarta. Your first stressful encounter will be overcoming your own inertia and faithfully keeping a food diary, then setting goals and letting others see them. But this should immediately produce some positive feedback. Believe me, the people around you will be just as positive.

Support Groups

I am often invited to speak before groups of people afflicted with arthritis. These people, often young, have a debilitating illness that medication often makes worse. It makes high blood pressure seem easy in comparison. In fact, because of the medication they use, many of them often develop high blood pressure to go with the crippling disease they already have. By supporting each other, they can bring help and hope where it doesn't always exist. Why not with high blood pressure?

I can't think of better support for people with high blood pressure than to take up a program of gourmet cooking without salt following Eleanor Brenner's book. Alternatively, the group could exchange ideas for pursuing a low-sodium, high-potassium life, or get together with an appropriate instructor for regular aerobic exercise. You'd be amazed how effective group participation can be at helping people succeed.

An added benefit of group support comes from the people you can invite to help you with your quest. Dieticians and home economists can give you all sorts of food advice and helpful hints. Doctors can explain in great detail many things about your illness and help you achieve a drug-free life. If you invite a physician to speak on dietary control of high blood pressure, you accomplish three tasks at once. The doctor learns about it and takes a positive attitude. You learn what he has learned, and through your questions you can force him to learn more and he'll be more supportive of diet and gain new patience. Each activity nurtures another. More important, you can learn how to deal more effectively with your own doctor.

A support group can help you identify new outlets and diversions. You'd be amazed how many people there are in this world with exciting hobbies and occupations. You'd be surprised at how interested and envious you could become when hearing people explain their lifestyles. Believe me, your mental wheels would start turning. In the end, however, the beauty of a support group is what the name implies: People with a common problem work together to help each other achieve a better life, and success becomes contagious.

Attitude

Make your motivation contagious. Use the thumbs-up concept and tell others around you how good they are. Send notes to people when there's something positive in what they've done. If a child brings home an "F," say, "I'm glad you didn't cheat," and go from there. Most people know when things aren't as good as they can be, and there's no gain in increasing guilt. It only makes it worse. Make the situation positive and inject some humor. You'd be surprised—it can become better.

Chapter Nineteen

Folklore, Modern Drugs, and High Blood Pressure

Unlike many chronic illnesses, hypertension, has not left an anthropological record. For example, arthritis affects bones and tissues so its history can be traced from skeletal remains, mummies, and frozen bodies. Blood pressure is not that way. There is no fossil record, and the well-preserved remains of a person with high blood pressure show no evidence even to an expert. To make matters worse, blood pressure couldn't be measured until about 1830 and then only rarely, by a cumbersome method. Blood pressure couldn't be routinely measured until 1906, and the folk remedies can't be traced further back than about 100 years. Therefore, we can't estimate effectively how much existed or what people did for it only 150 years ago.

This is in contrast to diseases like arthritis, gout, cancer, and heart disease, which have a rich history of folk and early medical treatment. For example, we know of effective arthritis treatments that are over 3,000 years old: similarly with gout and even poor eyesight. In two previous books, *Making the Vitamin Connection* and *The Arthritis Relief Diet*, I explained how history and folklore developed dietary remedies for many illnesses, even cancer.

High blood pressure is different. Societies whose diets have a K Factor of 3 and whose sodium intake is from natural food have at most a 1% to 3% incidence of high blood pressure, and about 90% of that high blood pressure is secondary to another illness. Blood pressure in those societies doesn't increase with age. In primitive societies that exist today, people over 65 have the same normal blood pressure, on average, as young people. So, until people started eating highly processed food with its K Factor of less than 2, and until serious overweight became a widespread problem, high blood pressure probably didn't exist.

Folk Remedies

Folklore does identify people with high blood pressure as having a "flushed face." People get a flushed face on becoming enraged, and this flushing was attributed to "hot blood." These people were also identified as very corpulent, often with gout. People such as the Italians, who ate a diet rich in garlic, didn't get the "hot blood"; but gout from corpulence was so prevalent and debilitating that its sufferers were exempted from taxes. In contrast, corpulent Englishmen of the same time often were described as having "hot blood."

Folk remedies utilized garlic and onions for the treatment of hot blood. Garlic has been used therapeutically in folklore to cure "hot blood." People who consume lots of garlic-rich foods generally have low blood pressure. These same people consumed a diet rich in soluble forms of dietary fiber. This fiber, as discussed in Chapter Ten, has a blood-pressure-lowering effect. Serious medical research of the last five years has confirmed that materials in garlic and similar bulbs reduce high blood pressure.

Garlic was used by Egyptian physicians in 1500 B.C. as a remedy for heart disease. This use, continued by Hippocrates (circa 450 B.C.), probably evolved because garlic lowers blood fats, most noticeably cholesterol. Although its effects on blood pressure were unknown in 1500 B.C., I speculate that it helped. I base this on the observation that heart disease was most often seen in seriously overweight people in those days. And of course, serious overweight is always associated with high blood pressure, even with a high K Factor.

In China, folk remedies are found for just about every human condition. High blood pressure is no different, and three herbal remedies persist to this day. Barks from the tree peony, philodendron, and skullcap root were prescribed by Chinese herbalists for high blood pressure. Unlike garlic, no studies have confirmed or refuted the wisdom of these remedies. These same remedies are still prescribed by herbalists today.

On Caribbean islands "hot blood" was cured by a mixture of aloe extract, leaves from several plants, and garlic. Aloe contains some emetics and is still widely used for therapeutic purposes.

The drug reserpine comes from an Indian plant that was originally given to people bitten by poisonous snakes. The snake venom attacks the sympathetic nervous system, producing, among other symptoms, high blood pressure. This use of reserpine led to identification of an effective cure for high blood pressure that results from sympathetic nervous stimulation. This approach is used today with modern, more sophisticated drugs called beta blockers.

Modern Treatment

Blood pressure measurement began in the early eighteenth century when an English clergyman Stephen Hales, learned to measure blood pressure in farm animals. He inserted a metal tube into a main artery, hooked it to a vertical glass tube, and measured the height of the blood. It reached nine feet with horses and was obviously unacceptable for human use, but this was the first step.

About 100 years later, in 1828, Jean Poiseuille, an ingenious French medical student, hooked the tube to another U-shaped closed tube containing mercury. In this way, the weight of the mercury kept the blood from rising very high. Poiseuille took his measurements in millimeters of mercury; the units persist today. In 1896, Dr. Scipione Riva-Rocci, an Italian physician, developed the ingenious idea of placing a cuff around the arm and pumping it with air until the pulse at the wrist was cut off. Cutting off the pulse gave the systolic blood pressure.

A Russian physician, Nicolai Korotkoff, brought blood pressure measurements into the modern era in 1905 when he placed a stethoscope just below the cuff devised by Riva-Rocci. He pumped to a 20-millimeter excess, slowly released pressure in the cuff, and listened for two sets of sounds, appropriately named the Korotkoff sounds. You should recognize the first sound as the thump, thump, thump of the blood just starting to come through as the cuff pressure matches the systolic pressure, and the second sound as the continuous "swish" of the diastolic flow, the constant baseline pressure of the entire system.

This brief 100-year history is hard to fathom in 1989, when you can purchase electronic sphygmomanometers in drugstores, discount stores, electronic shops, and even supermarkets. What's more surprising is the approach to treating blood pressure.

We might assume today that the records kept by the Janeways in 1910, showing that people with higher than average blood pressure died sooner, would have had the medical profession scurrying for a treatment. Not so. At the time, physicians rationalized that elevated blood pressure was the body's way of compensating for poor blood flow through the kidneys, so the Janeways' observations were passed off as interesting but not important until 1934, when Dr. Irwin Page did the simple experiment of testing blood flow through kidneys of hypertensive patients before and after lowering their blood pressure with drugs. At the time, his revolutionary findings demonstrated clearly that there was no difference in blood flow before and after. So much for the dogma of the time, but the modern era of treatment still did not dawn.

In the 1950s, epidemiologists conclusively confirmed the Janeways' less sophisticated observations that people with essential hypertension died prematurely. This convinced everyone that even mild essential hypertension should be treated and lowered as a life-prolonging measure.

Dogma in medicine is like dogma in any human institution. In 1856, a German physician, Ludwig Traub, had taught that high blood pressure was necessary for survival in some people due to impaired blood flow through their kidneys. It wasn't until Dr. Page did his simple experiment, 78 years later, that Traub's concept was proved to be a medically bankrupt notion. But it took about 16 more years for physicians to get serious about high blood pressure.

The first treatments followed Dr. Page's original experiment, which used diuretics to treat high blood pressure. A diuretic does what its name implies: It causes the patient to produce and eliminate more urine. Lots of sodium is expelled in the urine, so the blood pressure is reduced. A serious side effect is the loss of potassium as a normal component of urine. At first this led to a recommendation that people with high blood pressure eat lots of potassium-rich bananas. Later, potassium supplements were recommended. Diet therapy was not a dominant factor in the process.

Diet therapy began in the early 1930s with low-sodium, potassium-supplemented diets. These studies showed that dietary intervention could lower high blood pressure. In 1940, the famous Kempner rice diet study was conducted on hypertensives. This very bland diet, which emphasized rice, provided less than 500 milligrams of sodium daily and had a K Factor over 15. Therefore, it was similar to modern dietary approaches. In retrospect, the diet was bland, inadequate in many nutrients, but effective in reducing high blood pressure. It was a milestone in diet therapy because it proved conclusively that high blood pressure could be controlled by diet.

As I indicated in previous chapters, I had the privilege of knowing Dr. Louis Dahl, who advocated dietary control of high blood pressure. He developed a strain of rats that had hereditary high blood pressure; he was involved in extensive studies on animals and human volunteers that provided conclusively that essential hypertension could be eliminated in most people and extensively reduced in the rest. Since Dahl, many serious researchers and clinicians have controlled high blood pressure by diet alone. Indeed, people have returned to normal productive lives by following a high–K Factor, low-sodium diet program like the one in this book. These findings are so clear that the 1984 government report advised that diet should be a major first effort for everyone with high blood pressure, especially for people who, even when following serious dietary programs, still require medication. Although dietary control continues to demonstrate its effectiveness, the major treatment continues to be drug therapy.

Drug Therapy

When it finally became accepted in the 1950s that hypertension seriously reduced life expectancy, drug therapy was the first choice of treatment. This shouldn't come as a surprise. After all, during World War II, antibiotics had proven that drugs could work "miracles"; and to a large extent they could. As mentioned previously, the first drugs used were diuretics. As blood pressure became better understood, the methods of drug therapy became more sophisticated. Today, by government policy, a stepped trial-and-error procedure is used for each patient to find the mildest drug program that will effectively control high blood pressure. This approach helps to keep the drug side effects, which can be considerable, to a minimum.

Consider "side effects" for a moment. Any drug is a

physiologically active material that influences the function
of at least one and usually several bodily organs and tissues. For example, the most widely used drug, aspirin,
relieves most minor pain from headache or inflammation
by stopping the production of one of the prostaglandins. It
also exerts other effects on the stomach, however, so that a
person loses about one or two teaspoons of blood from
each aspirin. This side effect, loss of blood, goes unnoticed
until a person needs to take many aspirin and gets an ulcer
or colitis.

I had a sobering experience while writing *The Arthritis
Relief Diet*. A drug was being tested in our area that seemed
to have great promise. I even mentioned this research in
the book. Between the manuscript preparation and editing,
the drug was withdrawn because its side effect was too
severe: People died. That's the ultimate side effect, and it's
an extreme example of why your physician and the government policy move slowly and work up to the strongest
drugs. A continuing effort should aggressively include diet
and a constant effort to reduce drug use as the diet
progresses.

Nowadays, drug therapy in most cases begins with a diuretic, progresses to drugs that inhibit the sympathetic nervous system, then to the vasodilators. Each upward progression
of drug therapy deals with an increasingly complex system
and introduces more serious side effects. It is worthwhile to
consider each type of drug.

Diuretics

Diuretics cause the kidneys to produce a larger volume
of urine and excrete sodium as sodium chloride—salt. Therefore, diuretics work in two ways: One is to reduce fluid
volume by eliminating sodium and the other is to increase
the potassium–sodium ratio in the blood and reduce peripheral resistance. Both these mechanisms reduce blood
pressure.

Most recent diuretic therapies consist of two diuretics. This approach contains a diuretic to increase urine volume and sodium output, and another that spares potassium. These newer diuretics, in principle, have the best of two worlds, but it doesn't always work that way.

Side effects of diuretics consist primarily of excessive potassium and water loss. Ironically, one major cause of essential hypertension is a diet excessive in sodium and lacking in potassium. And a significant loss of potassium can have fatal consequences. Therefore, when diuretics are prescribed, the patient should be told to eat potassium-rich foods and use potassium supplements—basically to follow the diet in this book.

Magnesium loss increases from diuretics and can result in reduced magnesium levels. Since American diets are usually inadequate in magnesium, it seems prudent to also take a supplement of at least 50% of the RDA in magnesium as advised in Chapters Ten and Eleven.

Potassium loss can be serious. In fact, the consequences of prolonged inadequate potassium in the blood are not thoroughly known. The known effects include impaired heart function, kidney failure, impaired carbohydrate metabolism, and others. Obviously, a person on diuretics should follow the diet plan in this book and eat extra potassium-rich foods.

If you get the feeling that diuretics have some side effects that even increase blood pressure, you're correct. Eliminating potassium and depleting magnesium help to elevate blood pressure. But the fluid and salt loss counterbalance these effects. A little-known, very rare side effect of diuretics is dehydration, and that raises blood pressure by excessively decreasing the blood volume. Other side effects include interactions with other drugs, dizziness, nausea, excessive sweating, menstrual problems, lethargy, and loss of appetite. These symptoms can be totally absent in some and excessive in others. Under any of these circumstances, your physician should be consulted.

Sympathetic (Adrenergic) Inhibitors

In Chapter Nine, you were introduced to the "fight or flight" concept. This is the response to external or internal signals that increase the activity of the sympathetic nervous system, causing the heart to pump faster and the peripheral resistance to increase. Sympathetic inhibitors use that principle. They come in two types: one to decrease activity in the central sympathetic nervous system and the other to relax the peripheral system.

Centrally acting inhibitors work at the source, the brain or the spinal column. These drugs aren't drugs of first choice, and are often used along with diuretic.

In recent decades, alpha and beta "blockers" have emerged. In fact, I've heard people talk at cocktail parties about the "beta blocker" their doctors have put them on. It's not unlike comparing scars from operations. Beta and alpha blockers are drugs that work at the peripheral level and block the nervous system receptors, causing peripheral resistance to blood flow to diminish. In short, the arterioles relax and dilate, and blood flows more easily. Some blockers help to reduce the output of renin-reducing blood pressure by a second mechanism.

Side effects often become more significant as drugs become more sophisticated, and these drugs are no exception. The common side effects include dry mouth, drowsiness, dizziness, and sometimes nausea. These side effects are not trivial. For example, add drowsiness and dizziness to a cocktail or two, plus an automobile, and you've got a fatal combination. In some cases, complications include sexual impotence, depression, and edema. Obviously, these blockers are "big league" medications compared to simple diuretics. A major responsibility of the physician is to match the patient to the drug or vice versa. Matching drug to patient is a trial-and-error process that requires excellent doctor/patient communication. The effects of these drugs are a major reason why diet should be a part of any therapeutic program.

In recent years, newer concepts have begun to emerge, including drugs that inhibit the entry of excess calcium into the blood cell (calcium channel blockers) and drugs to specifically inhibit renin release. Predictably most are effective on some patients and have excessive side effects on others. All these new drugs represent an increasing economic interest in the dilemma that exists in a society in which high blood pressure is endemic.

Economics of Hypertension

Modern estimates place the number of people diagnosed with high blood pressure at about 36 to 40 million, say 38 million. About half as many more don't know they have the problem, but will eventually find out the hard way. So the total is about 60 million cases of known and undiagnosed high blood pressure.

Now, assume that 37 million people are going to take medication for their high blood pressure. They will probably have more than one form of medication; for example, a diuretic and a beta blocker each twice a day. That's about 4 tablets daily and possibly an additional potassium supplement or two. Let's stop at 4 tablets daily.

Four tablets daily taken by 37 million people comes to 148 million tablets daily or over 54 billion tablets annually! Now, if all hypertensives could be diagnosed, the total use would increase to almost 90 billion tablets a year. Suppose the cost of the tablets is about 25 to 50 cents each; say 35 cents on average. That comes to an astounding 19 billion dollars to pay for drugs for people diagnosed with high blood pressure. One new drug currently being tested will cost about $1.50 per pill; you would take two each day. The numbers don't seem "real" at that point.

This hypothetical cost of high blood pressure medication would almost double if the diagnosis were more commonplace. And the frightening aspect of it all is that the numbers of people with high blood pressure will only increase.

They will increase because people continue to gain weight, eat more processed food with its poor K Factor, lead sedentary lives, and consume more alcohol regularly.

Plea for Prevention

It seems to me that everyone has to eat; therefore, why not eat foods that don't induce high blood pressure? As a card-carrying member of the Institute of Food Technologists, I know that something can be done. The same technologists who make products laced with sodium can make them just as good without added salt and with an acceptable K Factor. And the excuse many of them often give me, "That's what people want" ignores the concept of leadership. Take a lesson from the automobile industry: Detroit was putting out enormous chrome-plated gas guzzlers that couldn't get around the block without a problem. At the same time, small, fuel-efficient, reliable Japanese cars were gaining sales. Detroit laughed, saying the people wanted big gas guzzlers and didn't worry about quality. Well, they were proven wrong. So it will be with health. As people, we have got to demand prevention. I can word it more eloquently: Nutrition is preventive medicine and food is the vehicle of its practice. A society that can put men on the moon can produce food that is in harmony with nature and is still tasty!

Additional Reading

Joe Graedon's The New People's Pharmacy
Graedon, Joe, and Graedon, Teresa
Bantam Books, 1985

Feel the Fear
Jeffers, Susan, Ph.D.
Fawcett, Columbine 1987

Take Your Life Off Hold
Dreier, Ted
Fulcrum, Inc., 1987

Scientific Papers Concerning High Blood Pressure
Sacks, F. M., et al. "Effect of Linoleic and Oleic Acids on Blood Pressure, Blood Viscosity, and Erythrocyte Cation Transport." *J. Am. College of Nutrition* 6 (1987): 179–86.

Webster, P. O. and T. Dyckner. "Magnesium and Hypertension." *J. Am. College of Nutrition* 6 (1987): 321–28.

Haddy F. J. "Dietary Sodium and Potassium in the Genesis, Therapy and Prevention of Hypertension." *J. Am. College of Nutrition* 6 (1987): 261–70.

McCarron, D. A. and C. D. Morris. "Calcium and Hypertension." *Annals of Internal Medicine* 103 (1985): 825–31.

Whitecarver, S. A., et al. "Effect of Dietary Chloride on Salt-Sensitive and Renin-Dependent Hypertension." *Hypertension* 8 (1986): 56–61.

Breun, T. "Alcoholic Beverages and Coronary Risk Factors." *J. Epidemiology and Community Health* 40 (1986): 249–56.

Stamler, R., et al. "Nutritional Therapy for High Blood Pressure." *J. American Medical Assoc.* 257 (1987): 1484–91.

Books Concerning High Blood Pressure

The K Factor.
Moore, Richard D., M.D., Ph.D., and Webb, George
D., Ph.D.
Macmillan, New York: 1986.

Understanding Hypertension
Caris, Timothy N., M.D.
Warner Books, New York, 1986

Adrenal glands, 89
Adrenalin, stress and, 94, 95, 96
Aerobics, 276, 282
Aerobics Institute, 65, 277
Aerobics Program for Total Well Being (Cooper), 66
Age, 14, 15–16, 27, 293, 304
 exercise and, 66, 272–73
 weight and, 255–56
Airline food, 212–13
Air traffic controllers, 95–96, 98
Alcohol, 60, 72–75, 98–99, 253
Alcoholic beverages, 72–75, 76, 132, 173, 212, 265, 313
Alcoholism, 26
Aldosterone, 89–90
 -angiotensin-renin system, 89–90, 95
Aloe, 305
Alpha blockers, 311
Amino acids, 116
Anaerobic exercise, 277, 281
Angiotensin, 89
 -renin-aldosterone system, 89–90, 95
Aorta, 19
Appendicitis, 127
Appetite, loss of, 310
Appetizers, 209, 211
Apple Pie, 243
Arachidonic acid, 82
Archives of Internal Medicine, 22
Arteries, 18, 19, 84
 flexibility of, 21–22
Arterioles, 19, 28, 69, 83, 84, 90, 96, 311
 number and diameter of, 21–22
Arthritis, 123, 303
Arthritis Relief Diet, The (Scala), 127, 303, 309
Artichoke, 209, 211
Aspirin, 309
Asthma, 123
Astropulse, 45

Avocado, 209, 211
 Tuna Salad, 237

Baked goods, 123, 154
Basal metabolism, 261, 267
Beans, 116, 122, 200
Beef, 118, 157–59, 163, 194
Beef fat, 78
Beta blockers, 305, 311
Beta carotene, 185
Beverages, 173–74, 212
 alcoholic, 72–75, 76, 132, 173, 212, 265, 313
 fruit juices, 132, 133, 155–57, 212
 sodium content of, 133, 134, 173–74, 212
Bicycling, 66, 276, 277
Biofeedback, 294, 300
Bitters, 215
Blacks, 6
Blood:
 cells, 84
 cholesterol, *see* Cholesterol
 sugar levels in, 57–58, 59, 94, 95–96, 124–25
 viscosity of, 21, 22, 79
Blood pressure:
 cardiac output, 21, 270
 high, *see* High blood pressure
 measuring, 6, 20, 41–44, 284, 303, 305–07
 normal, 20, 23, 61–62
 total peripheral resistance, 21–22, 79, 83, 84, 90, 95–96, 103, 309–10, 311
Botulism, 130
Bowel function, 127, 272
Brachiotype, 258
Brain, 272, 311
Bread, 126, 127, 141, 153, 192–93, 210, 217–22
 Oroweat, 142, 153–54
 Pita, 220–22
 sodium content of, 132, 133–34

316